Y0-AGL-032

YOGA FOR CHILDREN

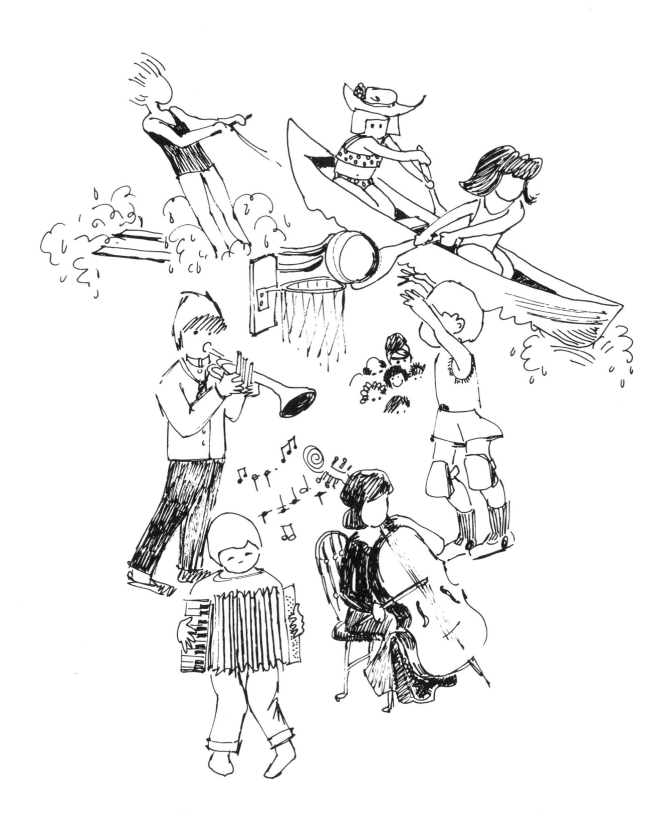

YOGA FOR CHILDREN

BY
EVE DISKIN

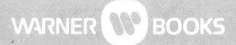
WARNER BOOKS

A Warner Communications Company

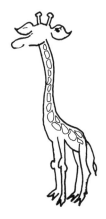

Copyright © 1976 by Eve Diskin
All rights reserved. Printed in the U.S.A.

WARNER BOOKS EDITION

10 9 8 7 6 5 4 3 2 1

Text design by Milton Batalion

Cover design by Gene Light

Cover photograph by Jerry West

Warner Books, Inc., 75 Rockefeller Plaza, New York, N.Y. 10019

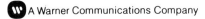 A Warner Communications Company

Not associated with Warner Press, Inc., of Anderson, Indiana

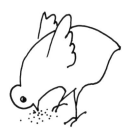

CONTENTS

ACKNOWLEDGMENTS

I am grateful to Frances Goldstein, who prepared all of the illustrations, which grace virtually every page of this book, and who provided many excellent ideas for the book.

For devoted and expert technical advice and assistance in shooting the photographs, I thank my son, Steven Diskin.

I also thank my friend Sylvia Shubert who helped me prepare this manuscript.

The contributions made by the directors, principals, teachers, and children of the following schools were considerable:

Alexander Montessori School—Beverly McGhee, James R. McGhee, Eleanor Winhold

American School for the Deaf—Kathleen Bannon, Dr. Ben Hoffmeyer

Arlette Salgado's Institute of Yoga, Neuchatel, Switzerland

Banzai Judo School—Lorenzo Mesa

Bel Aire Elementary School—Rosemary Brady, Louise Lockwood

Carrollton School for Girls—Sister Baxter

Cecile Appleton Academy of Yoga, Winchester, England

Chris Quirk Swimming School—Chris Quirk

Conchita Espinosa Academy—Conchita Espanosa, June McNair

Glen Jones School of Fashion Arts—Mary Chapman, David L. Lambert

Junior Girl Scout Troup 361—Jane Deacon, Jennie Tolson, Pat Miller

Marco Beach Hotel and Villas—Roger Everingham, Diane Weaver, yoga director

Ransom Everglades School—Frank Brogan, Cav Cavanaugh, athletic director

The Wesley Studio of Acrobatic and Dance—Wesley E. Stout, Tillman B. Williams

Ruth Williams School of Yoga—Ruth Williams

The children who posed for individual pictures have my full appreciation. They are: Frances Almeida, Karin Biarbeznt, Padenland Biarbeznt, Jill Bellins, Christi Chapman, Jennifer Cogen, Anthony Freedman, Marina Freedman, Kim Friesen, Ali Garcia, Jamie Goldstein, Jennifer Goldstein, Jessica Goldstein, Carlotta Junger, Sebastian Junger, Todd Kim, Yang Kim, Larry Kritcher, Kim Lavin, David Latson, H. Baird Lobree, John Lorray, Melissa Loshusan, Chandra Morgan, Rip Myers, Rory Myers, Arun Pathy, Nina Pathy, Eric Patterson, Geetha Rangachari, Jeri Rosenthal, Lisa Rosenthal, Kenny Steig, Karen Steig, Dawn Svaldi, Jo Ann Svaldi, June Warner, Pamela White.

The children not only represented the yoga postures like true little yogis, but remained patient and quiet through long hours of waiting.

I can say with much pride that every participant in this endeavor has, by his expression of interest and warmth, contributed immeasurably to that concept of life the yogis consistently live with and project toward others.

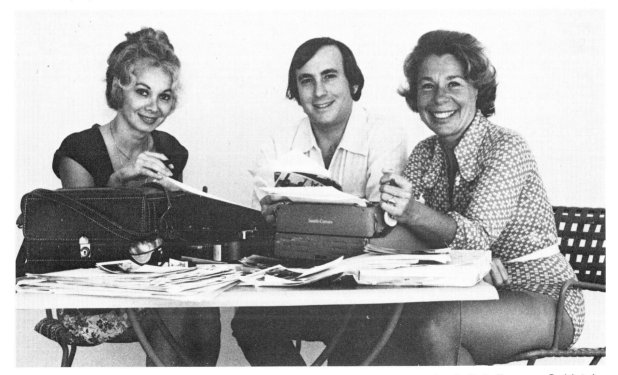

It took us a long time to put this book together for you. We hope you enjoy it. (left: Frances Goldstein, center: Steven Diskin, right: Eve Diskin)

I dedicate this book to Eugene S. Rawls whose love, wisdom, understanding, and direction changed my life. Through him I achieved a greater awareness of many things.

I also dedicate this book to D. Richard Sena, M.D., whose kindness and compassion during Eugene's extended illness helped us through many trying moments.

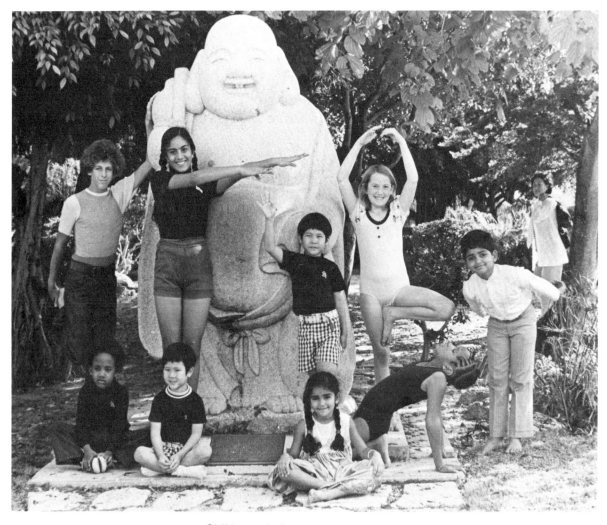

Children of all nationalities do yoga.

FOREWORD FROM A PSYCHOLOGIST TO PARENTS

For about ten years, I have been engaged in research concerned with the development of stable, close-knit family relationships that are based upon shared activities and values. I have been interested in building understanding among parents and children that would prevent their alienation from one another.

A child-centered approach to yoga is an exciting way to create healthy family togetherness. For approximately six thousand years, yoga has been practiced by individuals and entire families because of its positive physical, emotional, and meditative benefits, and it has the same potential for interaction today as it had in early centuries. Parents and children must have things in common to appreciate together, and yoga is an excellent shared activity.

Children love the attention they win from their parents for any proficiency they can demonstrate. If they cannot find something of real value to share with their parents, they will occupy themselves with anyone or anything to fill the void, irrespective of negative results.

Through yoga children are introduced to a healthy way of acquiring self-discipline and mastery in a variety of body movements. Self-discipline and mastery are words which evoke visions of constraint and hardship, but yoga can bring out both these capabilities in a recreational context, with no association of unpleasantness in the process. Yoga is particularly appealing to children because it challenges their "let me do it myself" spirit, and for its readily observable results. Even those children who fare poorly in academic pursuits can show achievement in yoga. The self-confidence they acquire from the accomplishment and enjoyment of their yoga exercises builds assurance in their approach to new challenges. Parents can do their part by giving generous praise and attention for each achievement.

Yoga can also relieve the tedium of idleness for a child whose activity must be limited because of poor health or a confining situation. Doing the Lotus Bud while watching television, for example, or engaging in the Balloon on an extended automobile trip provides a constructive outlet for pent-up energy. The child can be quiet without being unnaturally immobile or bored or feeling deprived of normal childhood activity.

I hope that parents everywhere will show approval when their children engage in yoga and will join them in it, both for its skill-building benefits and for its use as a means of promoting the kind of family interaction and friendship that are so necessary to a healthy stable home life.

Eve Diskin has, through her widespread yoga activities, played a considerable part in bringing yoga into the home and introducing it to both adults and children. She has shown that yoga is a salutary, effective way to share recreational activities. Watching my own children practicing yoga while their mother, Frances Goldstein, captured their joy and interest in the illustrations for this book has added to my conviction that Ms. Diskin's child-centered approach to yoga is one of the most inviting and reinforcing family-based activities ever developed.

MARK KANE GOLDSTEIN, Ph.D.

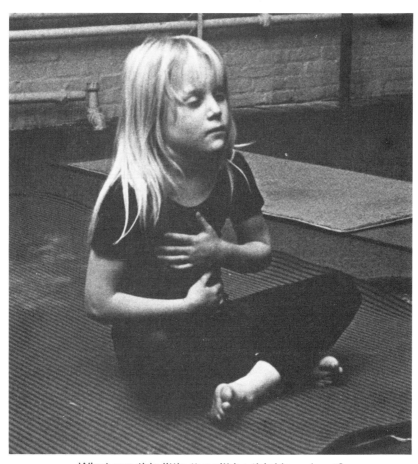

What can this little "yogi" be thinking about?

LETTER FROM A PEDIATRICIAN

The purpose of modern education should be a well-rounded individual—an individual with equal parts of brain and brawn. The ancient dictum of a sound mind in a sound body is still applicable.

Modern society seems to overlook the fact that there is an innate drive in children for physical activity. The problem is that older people forget the need, and do little to institute continuing physical education programs that complement the intellectual studies of school children on a regular basis.

Patterns of physical activity are formed in early childhood. They must be nurtured throughout adolescence if they are to play an active role in the individual's later life.

If the young child can be made aware of the fact that a sense of well-being accompanies physical exercise, and that it carries over into other aspects of his life, he will no doubt develop a wholesome respect for exercise. On his own initiative he will probably maintain the exercise pattern he has become accustomed to over the years.

I believe that a yoga book for children is a good way to awaken a child's interest in exercise. It is, at the same time, a doorway to mental development.

GEORGE Y. ELSON, M.D.
Pediatrician

PREFACE

For a good part of the fifteen years I have been teaching yoga, my classes consisted of adults whose average age was about forty. Then senior citizens (65 and older) became interested and joined my classes, raising the average age considerably. In the last few years, yoga has become popular with teenagers and college students, and they have attended my classes, too. Recently, parents started bringing their small children to class. This led me to initiate yoga classes exclusively for children. I was also inspired to write this book for children, all children, in their own language, to encourage them to learn yoga by themselves with little guidance from their parents or teachers. I realized that if these children could be brought up in the wholesome yoga way of life, they would have an opportunity to acquire and bestow on their generation the gifts of strength, flexibility, and serenity it must have if it is to deal effectively with the problems it is destined to meet. What they can learn from yoga now will be of inestimable value to them in keeping their physical and mental health on an even keel for the rest of their lives. I feel that the guidance my book *Yoga for Children* offers can be a priceless gift to a child from parent, guardian, or teacher.

EVE DISKIN
May 30, 1975

NOTE TO PARENTS

Dear Parents,

I am happy that you have selected my book *Yoga for Children* because I strongly feel that one of the most practical gifts you can give your child is good health, to which this book contributes.

If you encourage your child to make yoga a part of his daily life, it will soon become a natural routine. He does not have to master the techniques perfectly in order to have good results. As a matter of fact, it is best not to expect him to duplicate the photographs exactly, as his body has to achieve a certain limberness he may not yet have.

How many times a day does your child complain, "I have nothing to do"? Toys and ordinary games lose their challenge for him and bore him. Passively watching television for hours indoors neither improves his health nor his physical strength. Yoga exercises can help him develop grace, poise, stamina, and the power of concentration. Yoga exercises can safeguard his physical strength and his well-being by eliminating fatigue and recharging his energy. He can do them in rainy weather and in clear weather, indoors and outdoors.

Yoga can also give your child an opportunity to be with and to enjoy his playmates, as well as to be creative. Children can turn exercises into a fascinating game that they play together. Older children can help younger ones learn the techniques and the rules: They must not push or shove each other. They must never touch each other or roughhouse. They must never force or strain their muscles.

Yoga for Children helps to prepare children for a good life in a scientific way that does not conflict with any religious or psychological training they may receive. This way of life, which is based on ancient wisdom, is no less applicable today than it was in ancient times.

Yoga for Children is simple to learn and easy to teach, even for the child who cannot read. The book provides drawings and photographs that clearly illustrate the yoga postures. It also provides identifying symbols that are keyed to the names of the exercises. For instance, the Frog exercise is identified by the drawing of a frog. A black circle alerts the child to the fact that he is starting the exercise. A white circle tells him the exercise has ended.

Actually, the book needs little explanation because it is so simply arranged and illustrated. All you have to do is say to the child who cannot read, "Look for the picture of the turtle, the lion, the snake, the rag doll . . . Now, let's pretend that you are one." This will appeal to his imagination and sense of mimicry. He will feel that it is fun to imitate the different animals or objects pictured in the book. He can amuse himself by roaring like a lion, hissing like a snake, blowing out his breath like a balloon, and stretching until he is as flexible as a rag doll. By thumbing through the pages, he will quickly learn to find the exercises he wants because of the pictures at the top and the black and white dots.

Once your child has learned the basic yoga postures, he can use the techniques at school. For example, examinations often make a child tense. By doing, say, the first part of the Balloon exercise, he can relax. No one else in class need ever notice what he is doing. It takes only a few seconds, tension disappears, and he is prepared to respond to his examination with confidence.

Your child will probably be eager to learn yoga because it is interesting, but, if not, never force the issue. Try to motivate him so that he wants to practice the positions. One way is by attempting a few of the exercises yourself while he stands by to supervise. This will give you an opportunity to explain some of the new terms that he may find difficult to understand.

As a matter of fact, you might take time out regularly to practice yoga with your child. You would find that tensions disappear and minds become more alert than ever. Instead of scattering in separate directions after dinner, you and your family could stay together—building "togetherness" through yoga. Common interests tend to draw families closer, and yoga evenings could make pleasant memories for the whole family, for which, in later years, you and your child would both be grateful. Besides, yoga requires no complicated equipment, and during this period of inflation, when gasoline, movies, and baby-sitters are expensive, it provides a wholesome activity that costs nothing but a little time.

Please note: The suggestion that parents engage in yoga exercises with their children should not prevent the child who can read from going through the exercises alone, with his siblings, or with his friends, whenever he wishes. The book *Yoga for Children* has been written expressly so that he can follow it without help. He does not need your assistance in reading or in performing the exercises when he wishes to do them by himself and you have other duties. The child who cannot read should also feel free to carry out the exercises without your help when he wishes, once you have shown him the tiny pictures on the top of each page, the black and white dots, and the photographs and illustrations that illustrate the necessary steps. A little practice and the few simple, directing devices provided are all that he needs in order to recognize those exercises he can do.

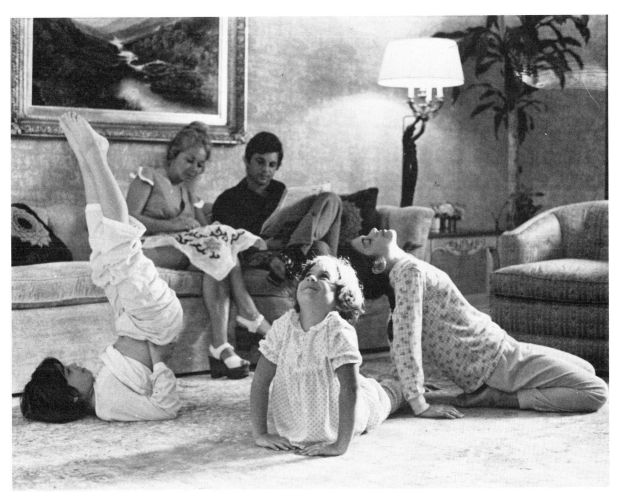

Mommy and daddy relax while the children do yoga.

NOTE TO TEACHERS

Dear Teacher,

Yoga is a scientific technique. You will find that your students respond to it with enthusiasm and interest, which results in general classroom cooperation.

Suppose you are faced with some children who cannot sit still. They fidget and squirm and race around the room. They fight with each other, throw things, tease the more docile children, and are impudent to you when you reprimand them. Soon you are ready to scream. It takes only minutes to do some easy yoga exercises that relieve class tension. On the other hand, you may find that during the waning hours of the school day, all of your students become tired and lethargic. They are unable to concentrate. A few yoga exercises can brighten their flagging spirits, raise their slumping shoulders, and loosen their cramped arms and fingers.

Yoga exercises are becoming more and more popular at every grade level—throughout the country and all over the world. While individual teachers in elementary schools are beginning to use yoga more and more regularly on a daily basis, many high schools and colleges have already incorporated it fully into their formal curriculum schedules.

Most yoga exercises take less than a minute to perform—some only thirty seconds. The results are immediate and the benefits lasting, and there are no sore muscles to cause discomfort.

The postures have such fanciful names as Rag Doll, Happy Feet, and Twinkle Toes. Children find the names amusing and the activities enjoyable.

The book provides drawings and photographs which clearly illustrate the yoga positions, and for the child who cannot read, it also provides identifying symbols that are keyed to the names of the exercises. For instance, the Frog exercise is identified by the drawing of a frog. A black circle alerts the child to the fact that he is starting the exercises. A white circle tells him the exercise has ended.

It is a good idea for you to do some of the exercises with your class; you, as well as the children, can profit from them. By observing your own reactions, you can gauge their progress. When you are certain that they have gained sufficient flexibility in the basic yoga postures, you can encourage them to do the more advanced exercises.

After using this book, you will discover that you have reinforced some of your teaching skills: the skills of calming disruptive students and of stimulating tired students. You will be influencing the physical and mental health of your students and creating an atmosphere of camaraderie in your classroom. There is no need to maintain a scheduled program. Yoga is an activity students can do in groups and as individuals, without the disturbing pressures of competition. Once you engage your students in doing yoga, you will reap the fruits of diminished stress, and you will note that a sense of well-being and closeness exists among the various student factions and between the class and you. Best of all, you will have the deep satisfaction of knowing that you are teaching young children a wholesome way of life that will benefit them for the rest of their years.

There is a great need for a national physical fitness program in the United States. The program should start when children are young. Such a program should include yoga. If every young child were guided into a yoga way of life, he would be well on his way to physical and mental fitness as an adult.

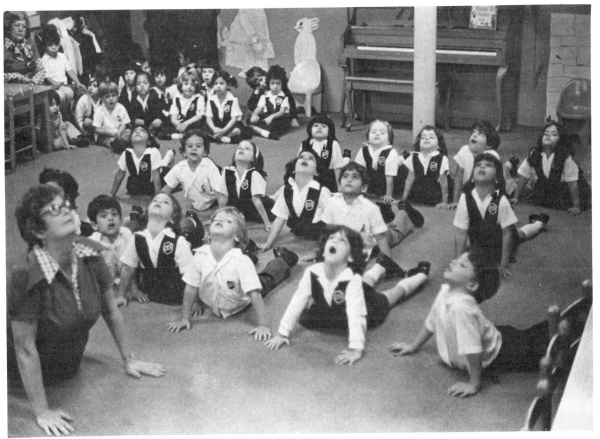

Kindergarten children love to do yoga. The ones in the back are waiting their turn.

WHAT THE UNITED STATES GOVERNMENT SAYS ABOUT GOOD HEALTH

In *Your Child from 6 to 12,* published by the Office of Child Development of the U.S. Department of Health, Education, and Welfare, in 1966, these comments appear:*

Healthy children have the physical equipment to make full use of the opportunities that come their way. They are more ready to learn, more skillful and joyous in play, better able to enjoy what is good in life, and to conquer what is hard.

Healthy children are also apt to become healthy adults. Their bodies grow better if they get enough exercise, rest, and the right kind of food when they are young. These factors also help them build up reserves of strength and energy for when they are older.

Now is the time, also, for children to learn about maintaining good health in the future . . .

. . . in our modern age, it is sometimes necessary to see to it that your child exercises actively. If you give your youngster the space and equipment for active play, he is apt to go along enthusiastically with an exercise program.

Your child is more apt to like this if it comes under the heading of sports and play rather than something that is labeled exercise.

*Chapter 6, "Your Family's Health," pp. 30–31.

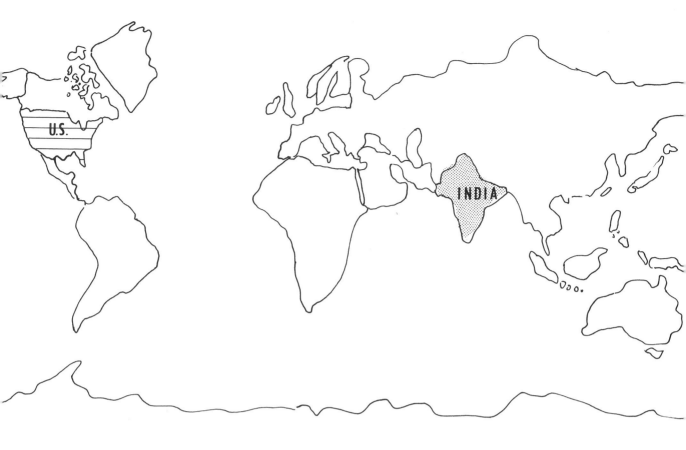

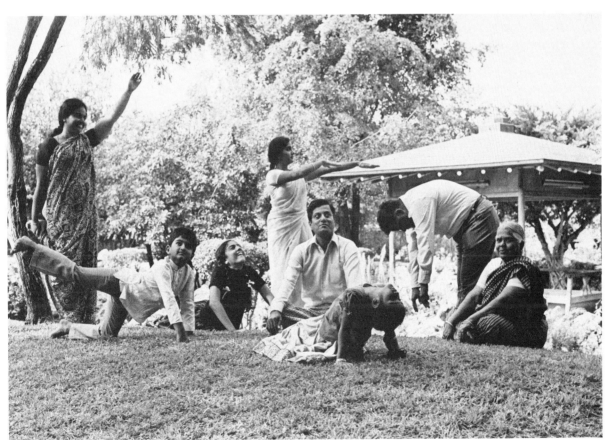

WHAT IS YOGA

Yoga started in India a long, long time ago. The name *yoga* comes from a very old Indian word that means joining things together. Some people in India began calling themselves yogis. They said that everyone has a mind and a body, and that the mind and the body should work together. They thought that if all people did exercise to make their muscles stretch, to fill their lungs with air, and to help their minds rest, they would be able to keep their minds and bodies healthy. The yogis believed that people's minds and bodies would join together to work for them—to help them learn what to do so they could be happy. The yogis also believed that people should put aside enough time every day to stretch their bodies, to breathe correctly, and to rest.

By watching animals, the yogis learned how to rest. Like the animals they learned how to sit quietly, without moving.

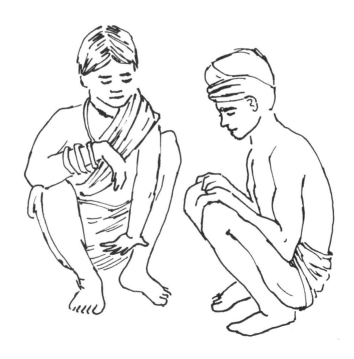

The yogis kept on watching the animals to learn more and more. They learned how the animals

stretched their bodies . . .

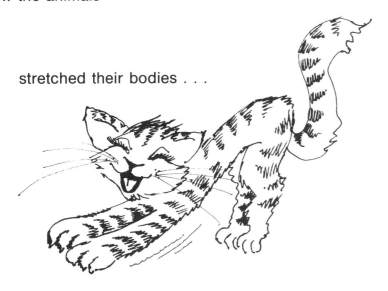

breathed with rhythm . . .

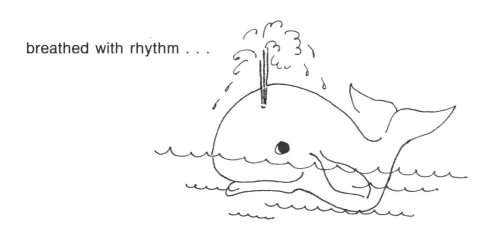

relaxed . . .

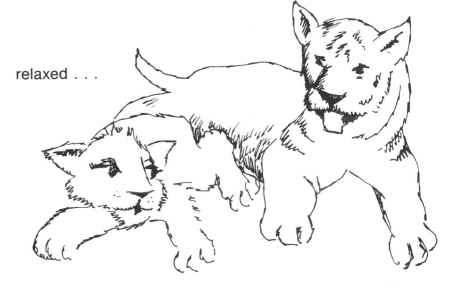

They copied the animals . . . and were able to stretch and breathe and relax too. They found that they could

swim better . . .

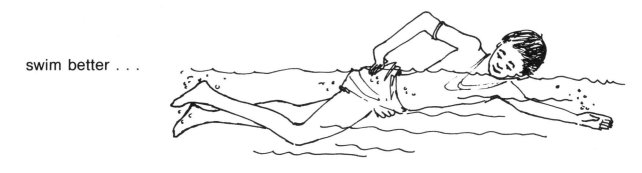

run faster . . .
and do many other things . . .

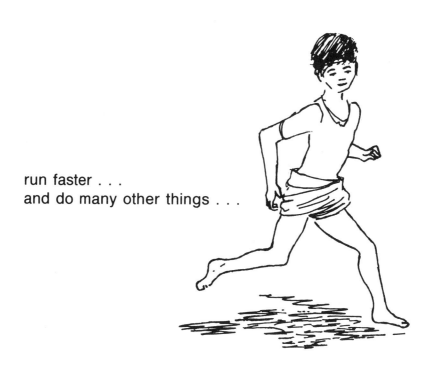

Their bodies grew strong from the exercises, and their minds did, too. The yogis liked to do the exercises, to rest, and to sit quietly and think because it made them feel good. It helped them to enjoy the world and to love the people in it and the birds, the trees, the flowers, the lakes, and all the other beautiful things in nature.

The yogis began to practice yoga all the time. Other people in India practiced yoga, too. Pretty soon people all over the world wanted to practice yoga. Fathers, mothers, boys, and girls began doing yoga. Of course, they could not do it all the time, but they did it as often as they could.

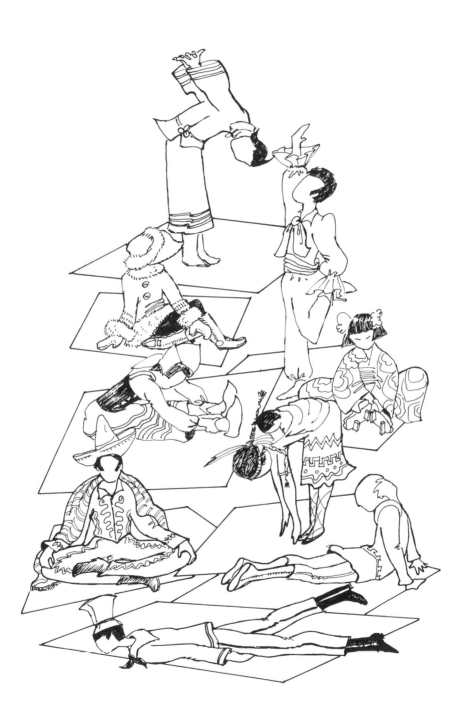

You, too, should do yoga whenever you can. It is not easy for you to go to India because it is too far away, but you can pretend you are a little yogi right here.

INTRODUCTION

Dear Children,

I am happy that you are starting to practice yoga. Yoga is easy to learn. Yoga exercises are fun. When you practice yoga, whether you are playing a game or doing the exercises seriously, yoga works for you. Yoga can make you grow as strong and straight as a tree,

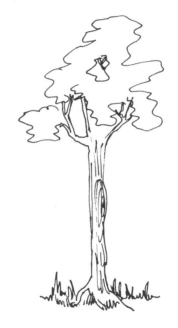

run as fast as a deer,

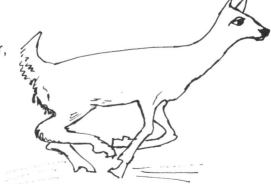

and think like a wise old owl.

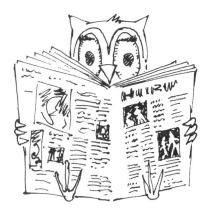

Wise old owls pay attention to good advice. Here is some for you:

1. Always practice your yoga exercises <u>slowly.</u> Don't rush. Take your time. When you are holding a yoga posture, count slowly.

2. <u>Never exercise on a hard floor</u>. Use a mat, a blanket, or a rug.

3. <u>Don't exercise after eating</u>. Wait two hours after a big meal and thirty minutes after a small meal.

4. Wear <u>loose clothing:</u> shorts, bathing suit, baggy pants, pajamas.

5. <u>Breathe through your nose</u> when you practice.

6. Never try to help your friends get into the yoga positions by pushing them. You might hurt them. Never let your friends touch or push you when you are getting into a yoga position.

7. Don't stretch yourself so far that it hurts.

8. You can do your yoga exercises out of doors, or indoors. You can also do it while you watch television. Once in a while, however, try to do yoga in a quiet place where no one will disturb you.

9. You can practice yoga at any time you wish: morning, noon, or night. But, try to set aside the same time every day. Before dinner or an hour or so before you go to bed is a good time.

10. Follow the book closely. Start with the easy exercises first.

11. Look for the black circle. It will tell you where an exercise begins. The white circle will tell you that you have finished an exercise.

12. The drawings will help you, too. They are always at the beginning of an exercise and almost always at the end of an exercise. They show you how to get in and out of the exercise.

13. In between the drawings, you will see the photographs. The photographs show the main part of the exercise.

14. There is something else. It is called a symbol—it is the little drawing at the top of the page that helps you recognize the exercise because it looks like the name of the exercise. For example, the drawing of a frog at the top of the page tells you that the name of that exercise is the *Frog.*

15. Ask your parents to help you if there is something you don't understand. Ask your teacher to help you if you do the exercises at school. Read the next part. It will tell you how to find the exercises you want.

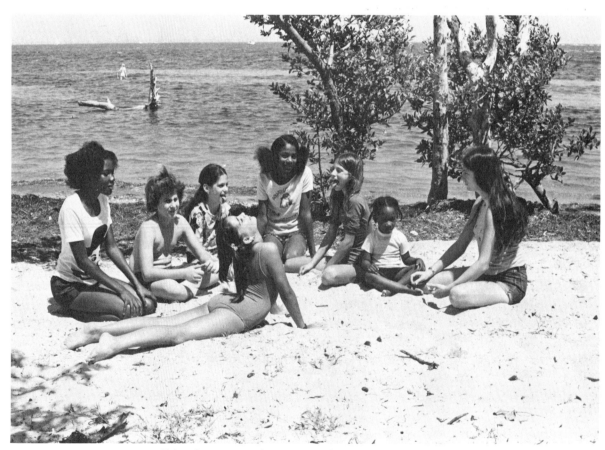

Friends get together to practice yoga at the beach.

HOW TO FIND THE EXERCISES YOU WANT

The first thing you should do is to look for the CONTENTS in the front of the book. It tells you where everything is.

In the CONTENTS you will see that the exercises are divided into three parts:

1. The easy exercises to do first—they are called BEGINNING exercises.

2. The exercises to do when you have learned the easy ones—they are called INTERMEDIATE exercises.

3. The hard exercises to do when you have learned all the others—they are called ADVANCED exercises.

On the top of every exercise page you will find a small picture. It is a picture of the name of the exercise. The picture changes for every exercise. For instance, if you want to find the Balloon exercise, look for a picture of a balloon.

The drawings and photographs will show you how to do the exercise. Every exercise begins with a drawing. The drawing leads you to the photograph. The photograph shows the main part of the exercise. Sometimes I say, ''Hold the position.'' ''Hold'' just means that in this part of the exercise you must not move. Any drawings you see after the photograph will show you how to get out of the exercise.

At the end of every exercise you will see a white circle. The white circle tells you the exercise is finished.

Near the back of the book there is a section called SPECIAL PROBLEMS. In this section you will find exercises to help you if you have a special problem like tired legs or poor posture.

Right after the Special Problems section of the book, you will find a page called an INDEX. On that page you will see an alphabetical list of all the exercises in the book and where to find them.

You see you have many ways to find the exercises that you want.

At the end of the book there is a page that will help you keep a record of the exercises you do every day. It is called an EXERCISE CHART.

Now you are ready to begin. Have fun.

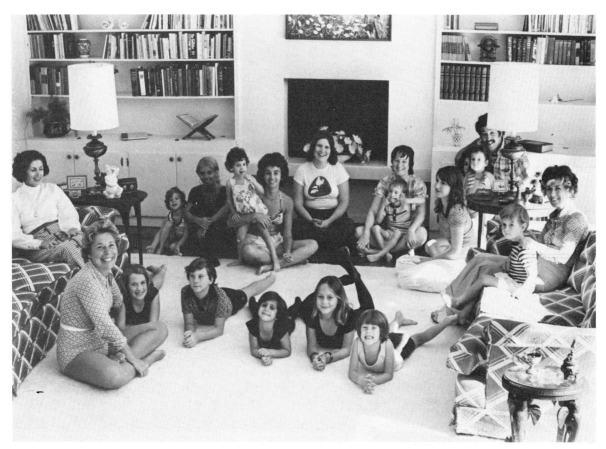

Come along children. We are about to start our class.

BEGINNING EXERCISES

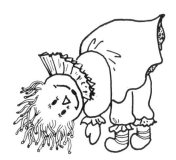

RAG DOLL

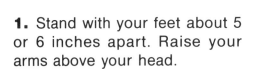

1. Stand with your feet about 5 or 6 inches apart. Raise your arms above your head.

2. Slowly bend forward as far as you can. Keep your head down. Hold. Count 10.

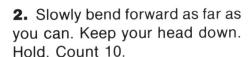

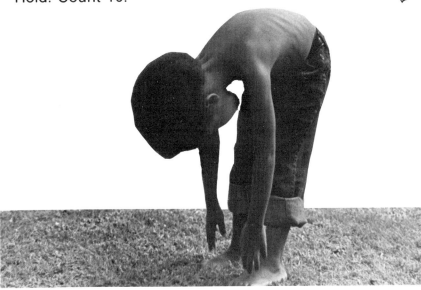

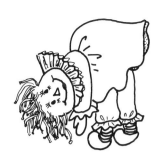

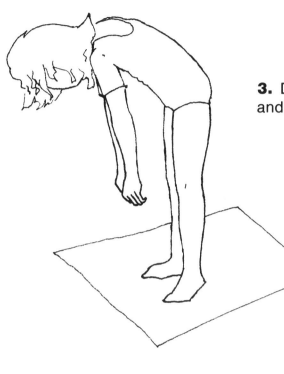

3. Drop your chin to your chest and straighten up slowly.

4. Hands to your sides. Rest.

HOW TO DO THE EXERCISE:

Be sure that you stretch forward slowly, come up slowly, and breathe slowly. Keep your eyes open, your feet wide apart. This will give you better balance. Try to touch your fingers to the floor. If you cannot reach the floor, just hold the position wherever you can reach. You should now be as limp as a rag doll.

After you have held the count of 10 every day for two weeks, try for the count of 15. Count 15 for four weeks. Then try for the count of 20. The longer you hold the exercise, the more slowly you must come out of it. Do the exercise twice.

WHAT THE EXERCISE DOES FOR YOU:

Wakes up your brain and helps you think

Improves your posture

Relaxes your back and neck muscles if they are tight

Gives you energy

NOTE TO PARENTS AND TEACHERS:

The Rag Doll is a wonderful exercise to do at any time of the day. It gets the kinks out. If children do it in a quiet atmosphere before they go to bed, it will help them relax and fall asleep. Just be sure that they do it slowly. If they do it in the classroom, they will relax and get rid of concentrated tension. They should be ready to resume their classwork in a jiffy.

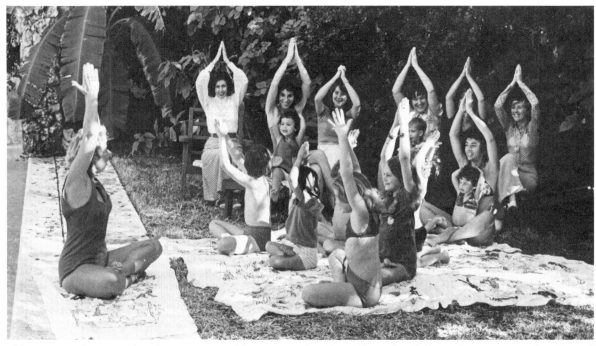

Yoga exercises are fun for everyone. You can enjoy them if you're little and you can enjoy them if you're big.

STRONG MAN

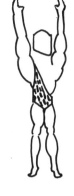

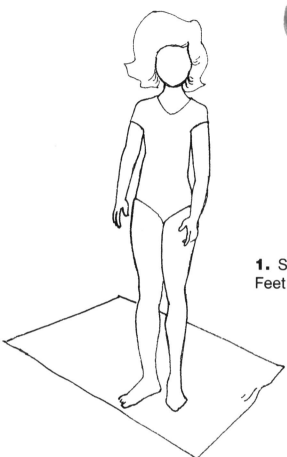

1. Stand. Hands at your sides. Feet apart.

2. Come up on your toes. Raise your arms over your head, palms together. Hold. Count 5.

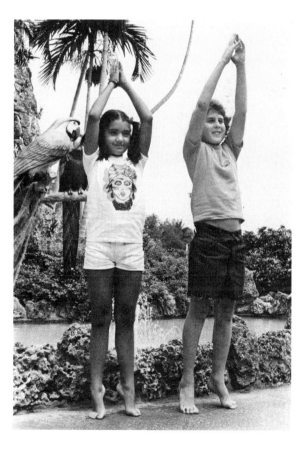

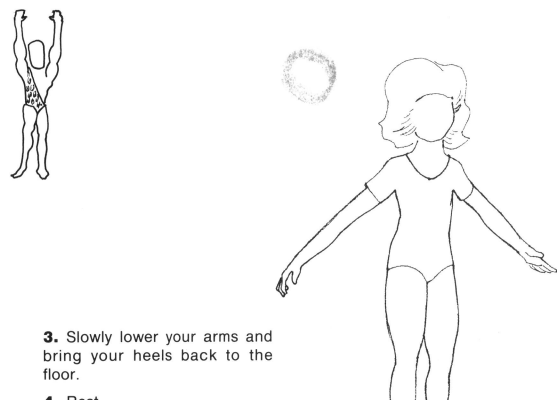

3. Slowly lower your arms and bring your heels back to the floor.

4. Rest.

HOW TO DO THE EXERCISE:

Bring your heels up as high as you can. Look straight ahead at an object that does not move. It will help you keep your balance.

After you have held the count of 5 every day for two weeks, try for the count of 10. Do not go past the count of 10.

When you can do this exercise easily, see if you can do something a little harder. As you rise up on your toes, take a deep breath and keep on breathing in until your hands touch. Hold for the count of 10. Then breathe out a little bit at a time until your heels touch the floor and your hands reach your sides.

WHAT THE EXERCISE DOES FOR YOU:

Keeps your toes and ankles strong

Helps you to balance

NOTE TO PARENTS AND TEACHERS:

This exercise tones up the muscles of the legs, making walking easier.

In the more advanced version, try to have the children synchronize their breathing with their movements. They should begin to inhale as they start to raise their arms and come up on their toes, and continue inhaling until their arms are fully raised. As they come down, they should exhale until their heels touch the floor and their hands are at their sides. It will probably take a few weeks of practice before they can adjust their movements to their breathing.

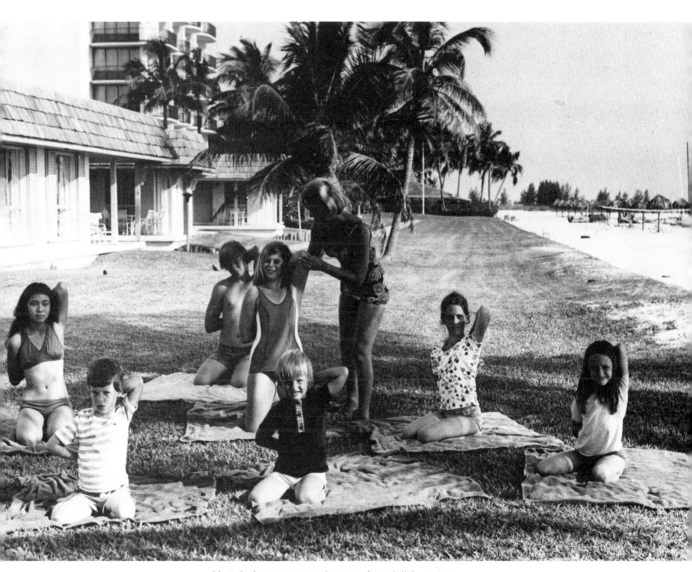

Hotels have yoga classes for children too.

KITTY CAT

1. Kneel. Hands on the floor. Raise your head.

2. Bring your back in. Hold. Count 5.

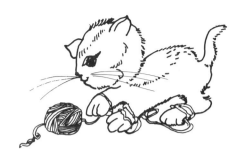

3. Lower your head. Push your back up. Hold. Count 5.

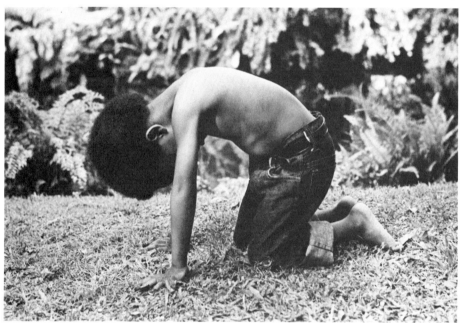

4. Sit on your feet.

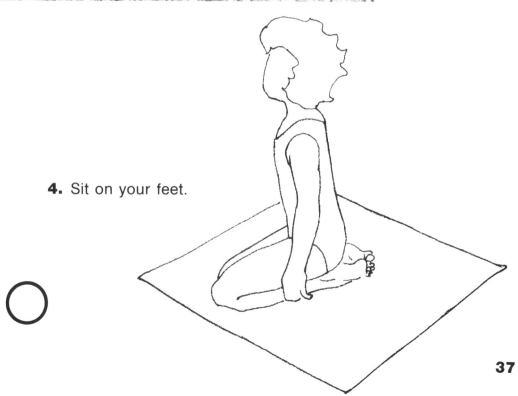

HOW TO DO THE EXERCISE:

Do this exercise twice. Do it slowly. Pretend that you are a cat stretching. Meow if you like.

WHAT THE EXERCISE DOES FOR YOU:

Makes your back and neck move easily

NOTE TO PARENTS AND TEACHERS:

This is a good exercise to do after long hours of sitting. It is a simple technique and yet it relieves cramped back and neck muscles. It also increases circulation to the brain.

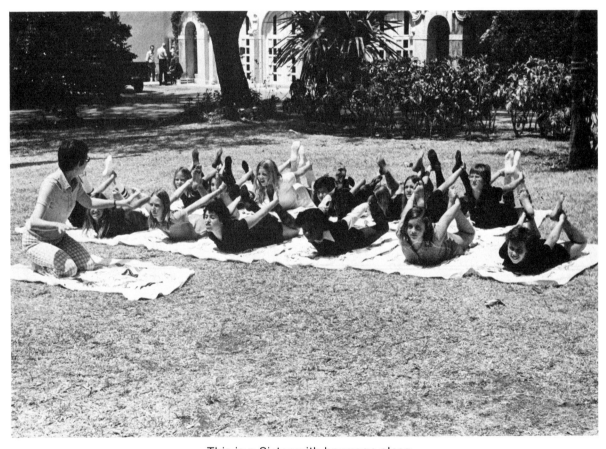

This is a Sister with her yoga class.

HAPPY FEET

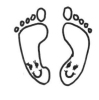

1. Sit on your feet. Hands on your knees.

2. Place your hands on the floor behind you.

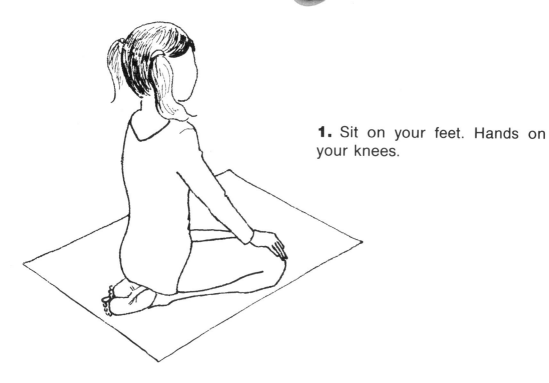

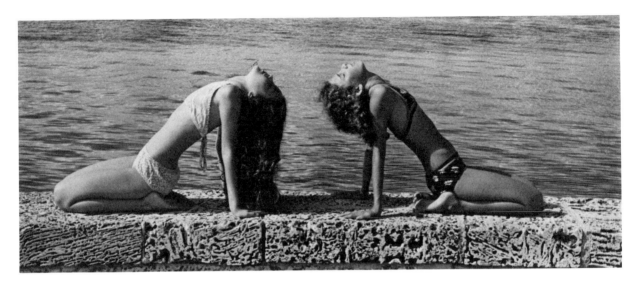

3. Drop your head back and push your back up. Hold. Count 10.

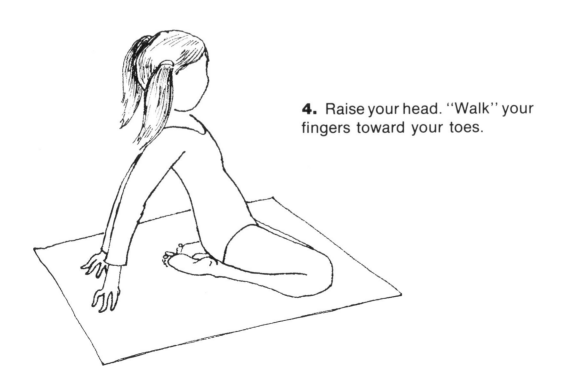

4. Raise your head. "Walk" your fingers toward your toes.

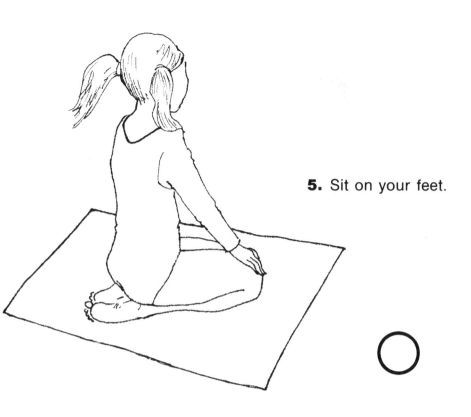

5. Sit on your feet.

HOW TO DO THE EXERCISE:

Practice on a rug or on the grass. If it is difficult for you to sit on your feet, do not put your hands behind you. Wait a few weeks before you try figure 2.

After you have held the count of 10 for two weeks, try for the count of 15. Count 15 for four weeks. Then try for the count of 20. Do the exercise twice.

WHAT THE EXERCISE DOES FOR YOU:

Gives you strong, healthy feet

Keeps your back and neck relaxed

NOTE TO PARENTS AND TEACHERS:

There are three yoga exercises that are especially useful for keeping the feet and toes flexible and healthy: Strong Man, Happy Feet, and Twinkle Toes. All three of the postures improve the circulation in the feet, which can be interfered with by confining shoes that prevent the toes from moving and gripping as they should. The Happy Feet position is a good one to sit in whenever children have some spare time, or even when they read, watch television, or talk with their friends.

GIRAFFE

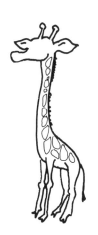

1. Sit at a desk or a table, or lie on the floor. Place your hands on each side of your face.

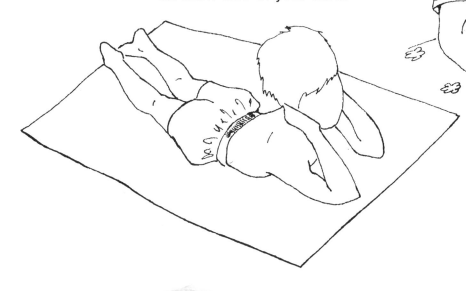

2. Lower your head and place your hands on the back of your head. Gently push your chin into your chest. Hold. Count 5.

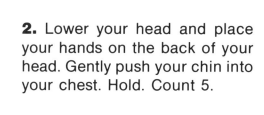

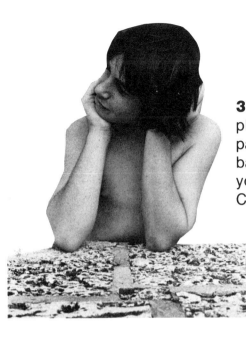

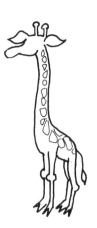

3. Slowly raise your head and place your chin in your right palm. Place your left hand on the back of your head. Gently turn your head to the right. Hold. Count 5.

4. Place your chin in your left palm. Place your right hand on the back of your head. Turn your head to the left. Hold. Count 5.

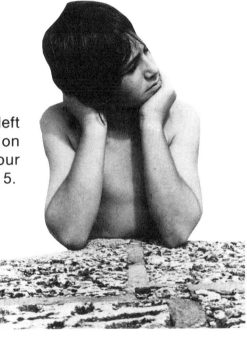

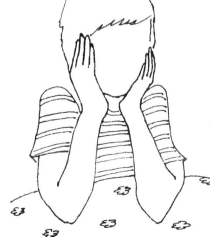

5. Look straight ahead. Place your face between your hands.

HOW TO DO THE EXERCISE:

Move your head slowly from side to side and push down gently. Do not force your head to turn too much to either side. Stretch only as far as you can.

After you have held the count of 5 every day for two weeks, try for the count of 10. Do not go past the count of 10. Do the exercise twice.

WHAT THE EXERCISE DOES FOR YOU:

Keeps your neck muscles relaxed

Helps you sleep better

NOTE TO TEACHERS:

This would be a good exercise for you to use in the classroom. It has a quieting effect on restless children.

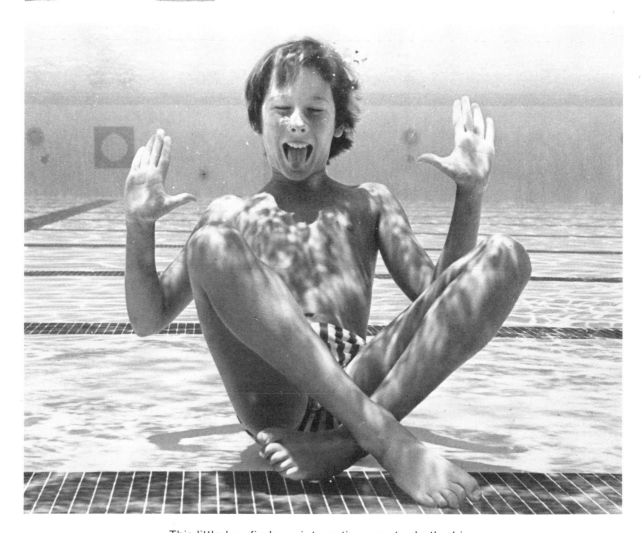

This little boy finds an interesting way to do the Lion.

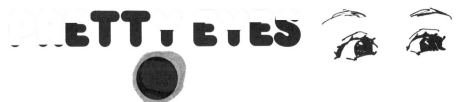

PRETTY EYES

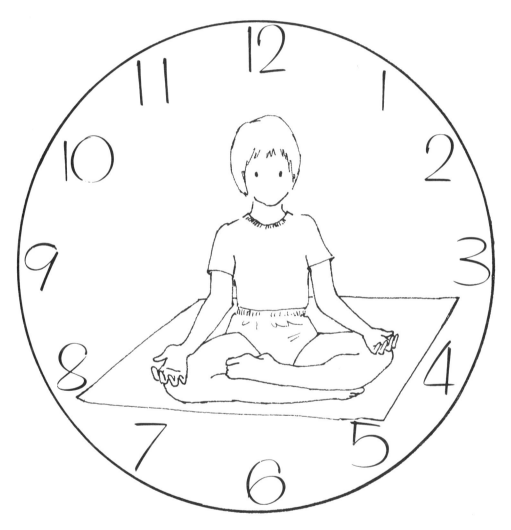

1. Imagine yourself sitting in the center of a giant clock.

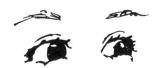

2. Look at the 12.

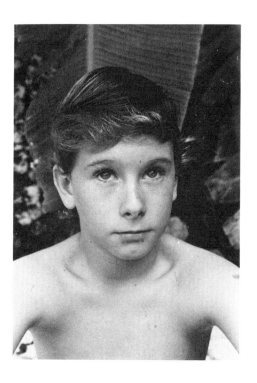

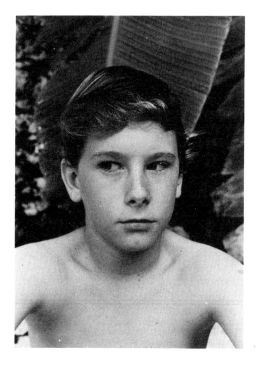

3. Move your eyes from 12 to 1 and keep going around the clock. See the numbers 2, 3, 4, 5, 6, 7, 8, 9, 10, 11, and come back to 12. Go around the clock 3 times. Close your eyes.

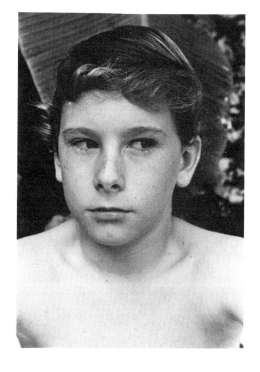

4. Open your eyes and move them around the clock going the other way. See the numbers 12, 11, 10, 9, 8, 7, 6, 5, 4, 3, 2, 1, and come back to 12. Go around the clock 3 times on this side, too. Close your eyes.

HOW TO DO THE EXERCISE:

When you move your eyes, keep them open as if you are really looking at a clock. Stop for a second at each number. Be sure you do not turn your head as you move your eyes.

WHAT THE EXERCISE DOES FOR YOU:

Helps to strengthen your eye muscles

Keeps your eyes from getting tired when you have to use them a lot

NOTE TO PARENTS AND TEACHERS:

Eyes tire from constant use. Exercising the eye muscles refreshes and strengthens the eyes.

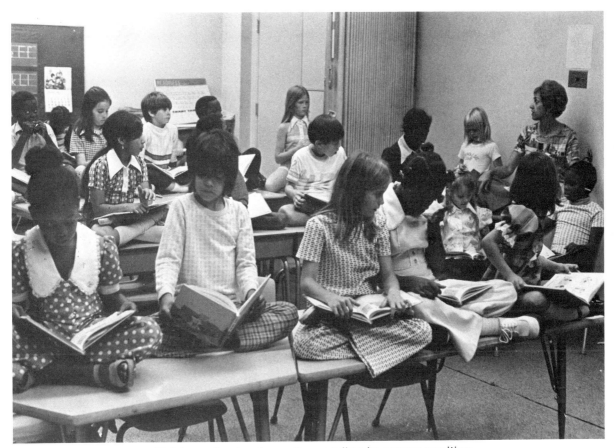

Children at school practice reading in a yoga position.

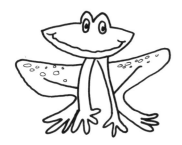

FROG

1. Sit. Hands on the floor. Bring your feet together.

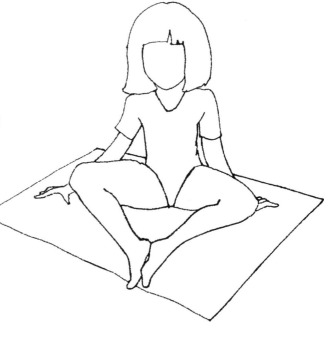

2. Place your hands around your feet. Pull your feet toward your thighs.

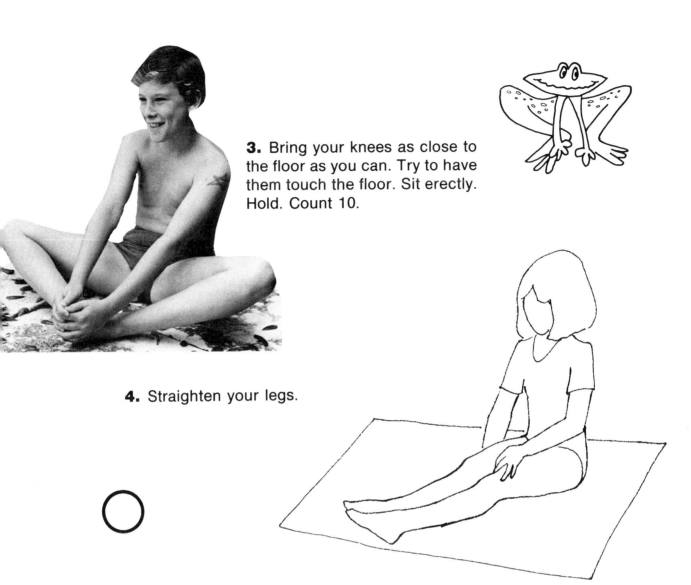

3. Bring your knees as close to the floor as you can. Try to have them touch the floor. Sit erectly. Hold. Count 10.

4. Straighten your legs.

HOW TO DO THE EXERCISE:

You must bring your feet as close to your thighs as you can and keep your back straight. It may take a few weeks before you can get your knees to touch the floor.

After you have held the count of 10 every day for two weeks, try for the count of 15. Count 15 for four weeks. Then try for the count of 20. Do the exercise twice.

WHAT THE EXERCISE DOES FOR YOU:

Strengthens your legs and keeps them flexible so you can jump and run easily

NOTE TO PARENTS AND TEACHERS:

This yoga exercise may look easy, but it is not. It often takes quite a while before some children can get their knees to touch the floor. Include it frequently because it stretches the legs in a way that no other exercise does.

SLEEPER

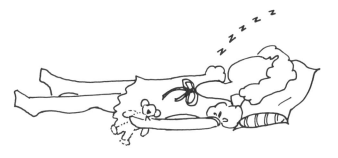

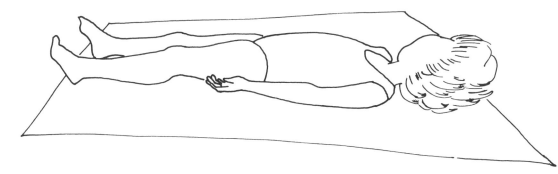

1. Lie on your back, legs apart, the palms of your hands facing up.

2. Close your eyes. Keep your mouth open a little. Breathe through your nose.

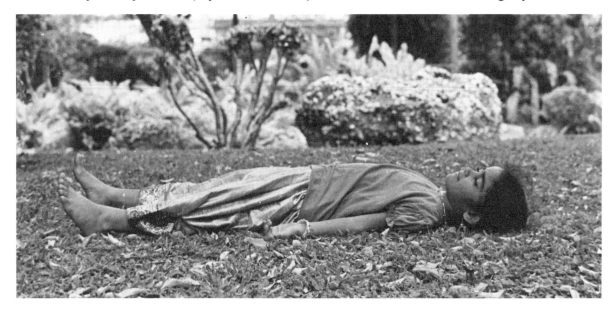

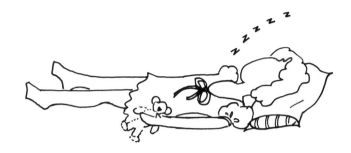

3. Make a fist with your right hand. Tighten your arm. Relax your arm.

4. Make a fist with your left hand. Tighten your arm. Relax your arm.

5. Tighten your right leg. Relax your leg.

6. Tighten your left leg. Relax your leg.

7. Tighten your eyes, nose, and mouth. Relax your eyes, nose, and mouth.

8. Keep your mouth open a little. Breathe slowly through your nose.

9. Relax.

HOW TO DO THE EXERCISE:

There is nothing hard about this exercise. After you have finished doing all the steps, pretend that you are sleeping. Do so for as long as you like. You need only do the exercise once each time, but you may do it as many times during the day as you wish. Be sure you are lying on something soft.

WHAT THE EXERCISE DOES FOR YOU:

Helps you to relax when you are tense

Helps you to fall asleep

NOTE TO PARENTS AND TEACHERS:

Nervous, high-strung children may have trouble relaxing at first. If so, tell them to concentrate on their breathing—they should inhale and exhale very slowly.

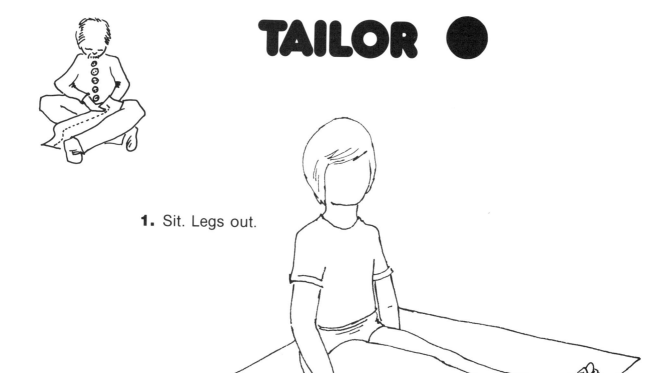

TAILOR ●

1. Sit. Legs out.

2. Cross your legs. Place your right leg under your left leg. Put your hands on your knees. Hold. Count 30.

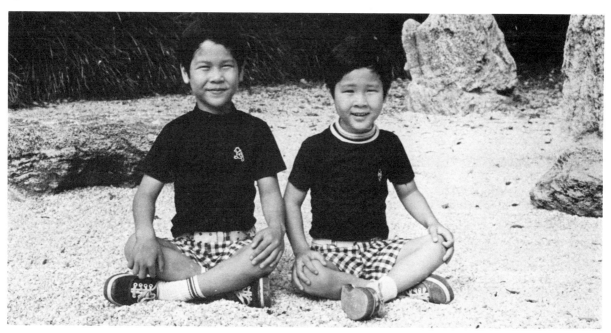

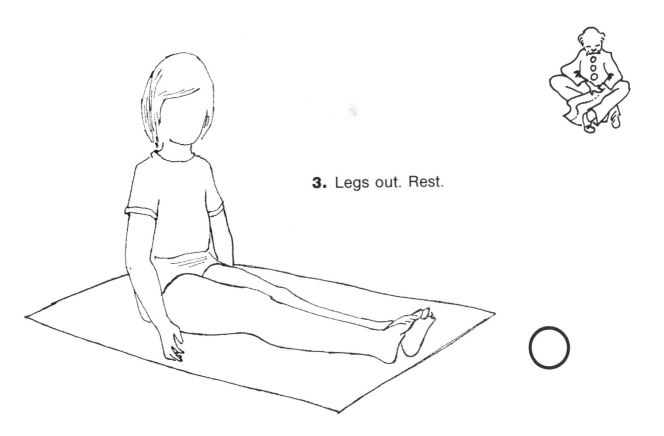

3. Legs out. Rest.

4. Repeat with your left leg under your right leg.

HOW TO DO THE EXERCISE:

Bring your feet as close to your body as you can. Try to keep your knees near the floor. Sit with your back straight. After you count 30 every day for two weeks, add 10 every week until you reach the count of 60. You may then sit for as long as you comfortably can. Remember to change legs.

WHAT THE EXERCISE DOES FOR YOU:

Helps you to run and jump better

NOTE TO PARENTS AND TEACHERS:

This is the simplest of all the yoga sitting positions. The child should start by sitting this way. After he has mastered the Tailor posture, he can go on to the Lotus Bud posture, and then to the Lotus Flower posture. As with all the other yoga exercises, do not allow him to force his body into these postures.

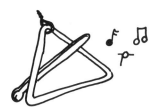

TRIANGLE

1. Stand with your feet apart. Lean to the right and place your hand on your right thigh.

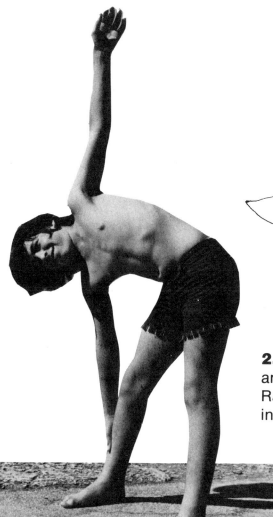

2. Slide your arm down your leg and drop your head to the right. Raise your left arm straight up in the air. Hold. Count 5.

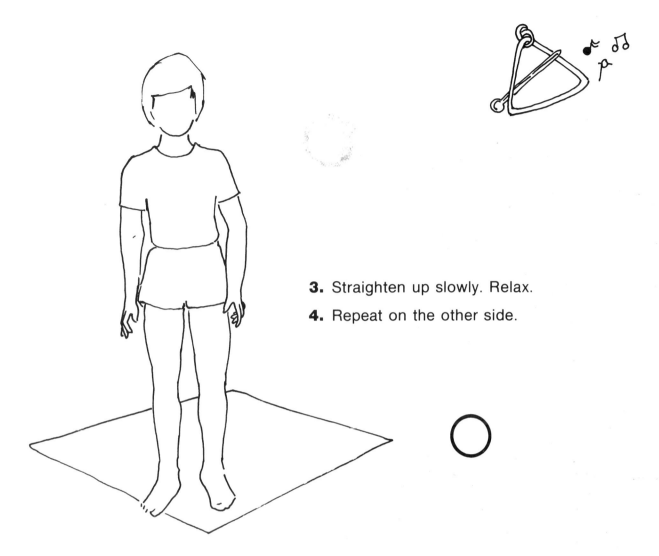

3. Straighten up slowly. Relax.

4. Repeat on the other side.

HOW TO DO THE EXERCISE:

This is a side stretch. Do not lean forward. Do not stretch too far at first. With practice you will be able to reach your calf and maybe even your ankle.

After you have held the count of 5 for two weeks, try for the count of 10. Do not go past the count of 10. Do this exercise twice.

WHAT THE EXERCISE DOES FOR YOU:

Keeps your sides and your back nice and loose, making it easy for you to move about

NOTE TO PARENTS AND TEACHERS:

This technique stretches the left and right sides of the body. It relieves tightness in the neck and brings blood to the head. It is one of the few yoga exercises dealing with a side stretch rather than a forward or backward stretch, and should not be omitted from any repertoire if coverage of all parts of the body is to be achieved.

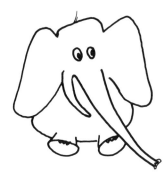

ELEPHANT TRUNK

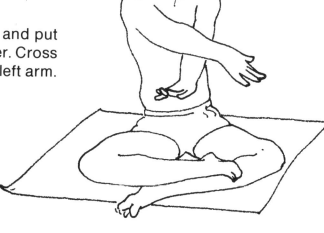

1. Sit. Bend your knees and put one leg on top of the other. Cross your right arm over your left arm.

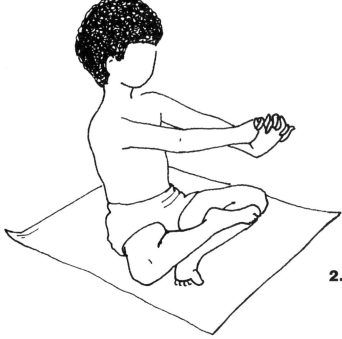

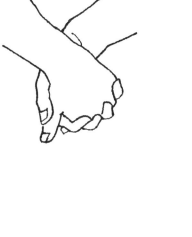

2. Clasp your fingers together.

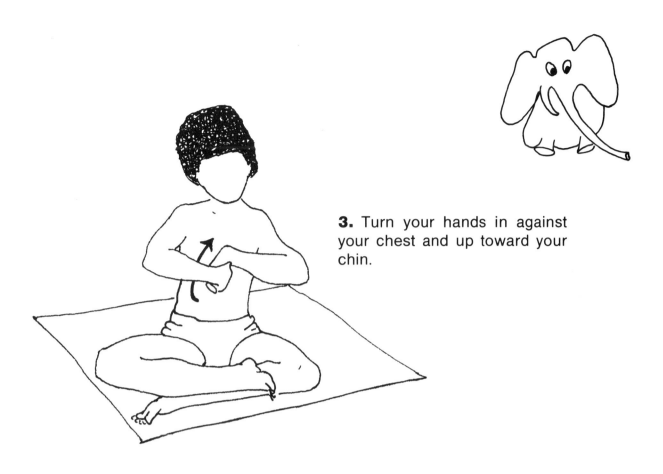

3. Turn your hands in against your chest and up toward your chin.

4. Straighten your arms. Hold. Count 5.

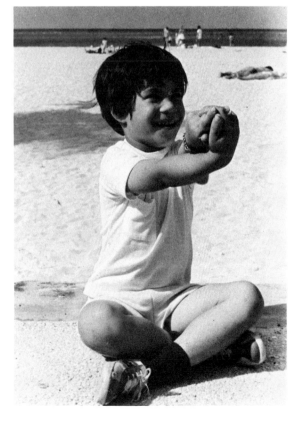

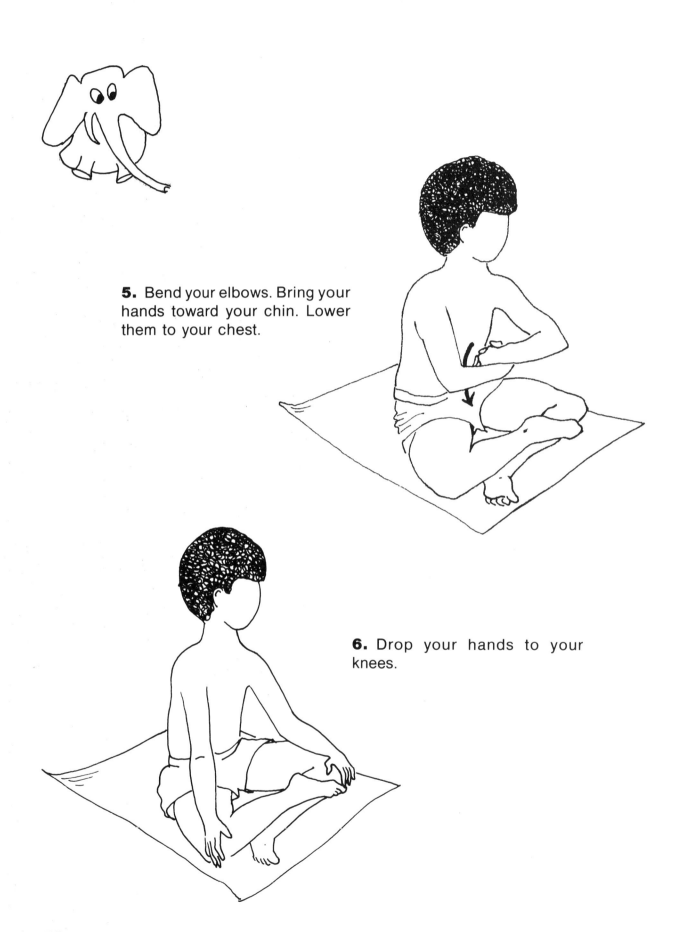

5. Bend your elbows. Bring your hands toward your chin. Lower them to your chest.

6. Drop your hands to your knees.

7. Cross your left arm over your right arm and repeat the exercise.

8. Relax.

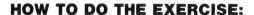

HOW TO DO THE EXERCISE:

If you find it hard to straighten your arms, loosen your fingers.

After you have held the count of 5 for two weeks, try for the count of 10. Do not go past the count of 10. Do the exercise twice.

WHAT THE EXERCISE DOES FOR YOU:

Makes your fingers move easily

NOTE TO PARENTS AND TEACHERS:

This exercise strengthens the fingers and keeps the fingers, wrists, and elbows flexible.

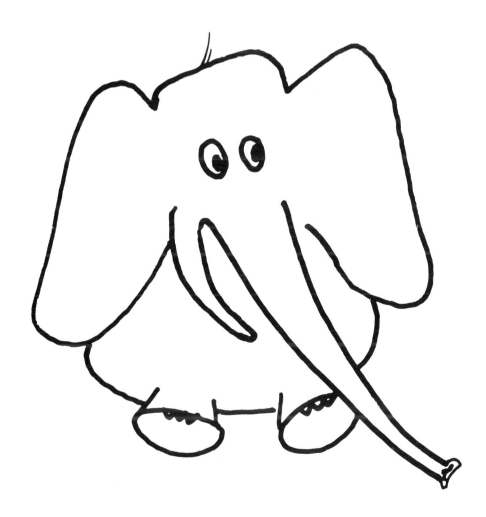

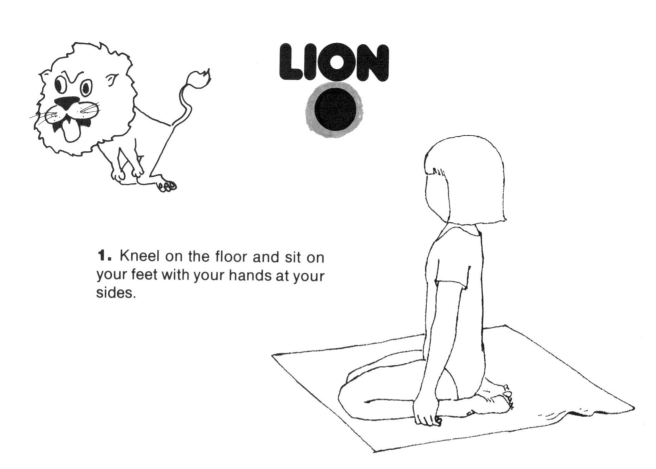

LION

1. Kneel on the floor and sit on your feet with your hands at your sides.

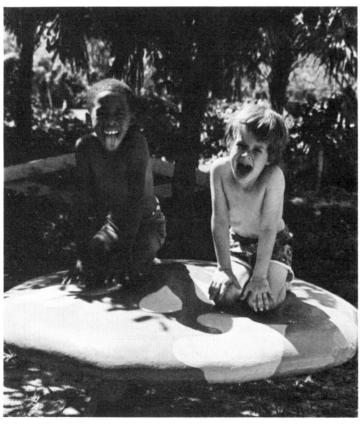

2. Place your hands on your knees and stretch your fingers. Widen your eyes and stretch your tongue out. Hold. Count 10.

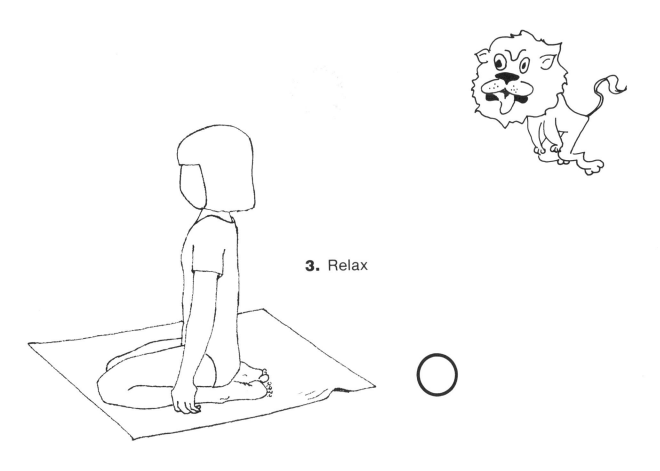

3. Relax

HOW TO DO THE EXERCISE:

Lean forward slightly when you do this exercise, like a wild lion about to spring. Bring your tongue as far out of your mouth as you can and try to touch your chin with it. Make all the sounds you think a lion should make.

Hold the exercise for the count of 10. Do not go past the count of 10. Do the exercise twice.

WHAT THE EXERCISE DOES FOR YOU:

Makes your throat feel good

NOTE TO PARENTS AND TEACHERS:

The Lion is a good fun exercise to do in school. Children can do it while sitting at their desks. It breaks tension and has an invigorating effect. Lots of giggles go along with it.

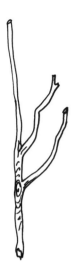

TWIG

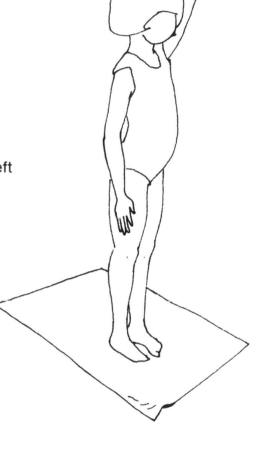

1. Stand straight. Raise your left arm.

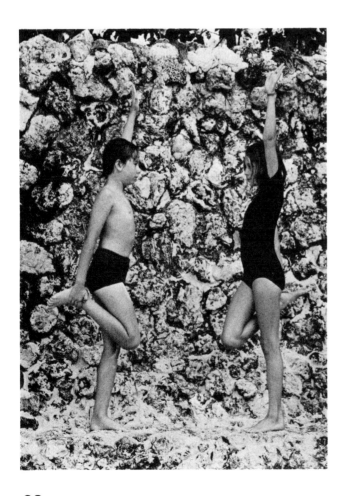

2. Grab your right foot. Balance yourself. Hold. Count 5.

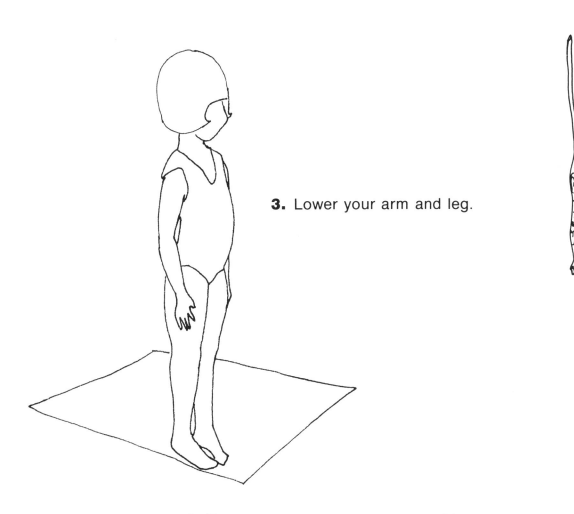

3. Lower your arm and leg.

4. Repeat with your other arm and leg.

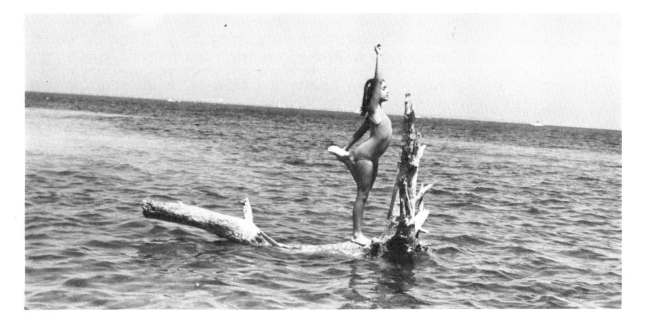

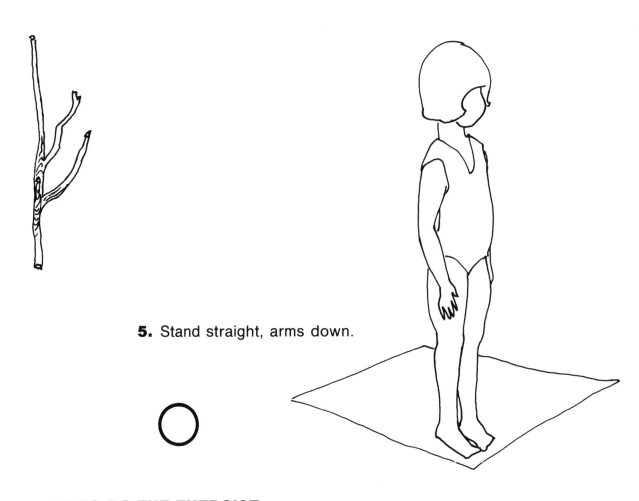

5. Stand straight, arms down.

HOW TO DO THE EXERCISE:

If you find it hard to get your balance, place your left foot about 3 inches from the wall and lean your left arm against the wall. Grab your right foot. When you feel that you can balance yourself, move your left arm away from the wall. You will have to use the wall again when you change sides. To keep your balance, pick out a spot in front of you. Keep your eyes on it. Looking straight ahead at something that does not move can help you to hold your balance.

Keep this rule in mind when you are holding the exercise: When your left arm is up, your right leg is up. When your right arm is up, your left leg is up.

After you have held the count of 5 for two weeks, try for the count of 10. Do the exercise twice.

Hold the count of 10 for four weeks, then try something more advanced. Let your arm and head drop back. Pull the leg that you are holding up as high as it will go. Repeat the same count. Do the exercise twice.

WHAT THE EXERCISE DOES FOR YOU:

Helps you to keep your mind on what you are doing

Gives you better balance

NOTE TO PARENTS AND TEACHERS:

Not everybody has good balance. Many children have to practice this exercise a number of times before they are able to stand on one leg without falling over. Once your children are able to balance themselves, you will find that they will walk and dance more gracefully and be more coordinated in their sports.

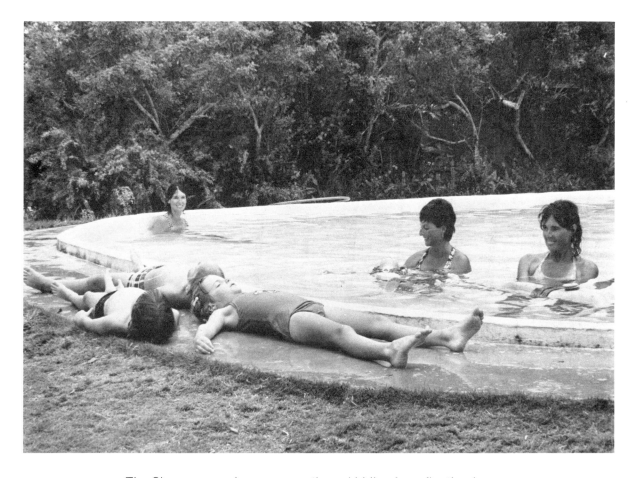

The Sleeper exercise prepares these kiddies for a floating lesson.

ROWBOAT

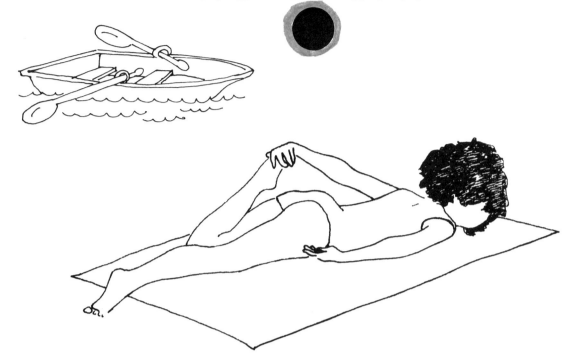

1. Lie on your tummy. Hold your left foot and gently pull it up to the outside of your thigh.

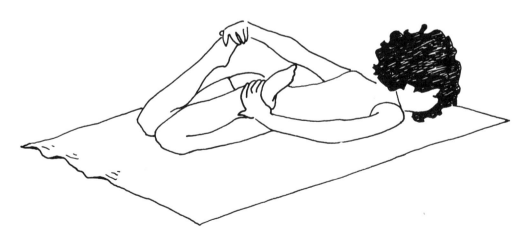

2. Gently pull your right foot to the outside of your thigh.

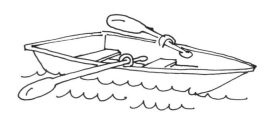

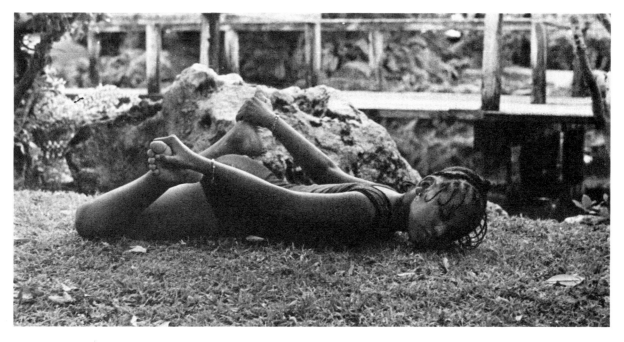

3. Push your feet closer to the floor. Hold. Count 5.

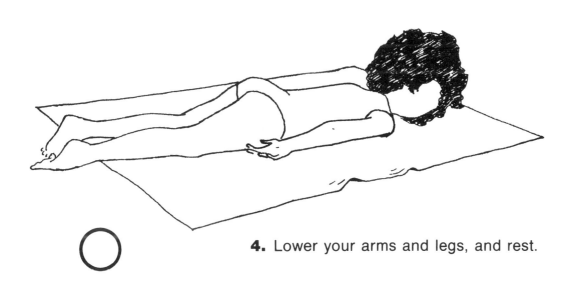

4. Lower your arms and legs, and rest.

HOW TO DO THE EXERCISE:

After you have held the count of 5 for two weeks, try for the count of 10. Do not go past the count of 10. Do the exercise twice.

WHAT THE EXERCISE DOES FOR YOU:

Keeps your legs strong and able to move easily

Stretches and strengthens your lower back

NOTE TO PARENTS AND TEACHERS:

This exercise keeps knees, legs, and ankles flexible, and is an aid to children who engage in sports. It is of general value in relieving tired, aching legs. In the photograph, you can see that the child's feet are far from the floor. Most children cannot get their feet close to the floor. With considerable practice, however, they are able to reach as close as one or two inches from the floor. The weight of their hands on their feet is sufficient to stretch their legs as they push down. Never let a child force a stretch.

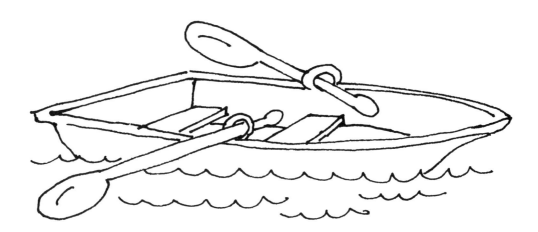

JELLY ROLL

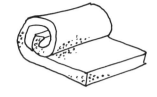

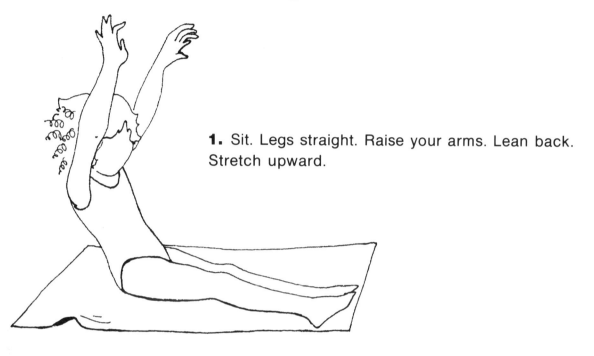

1. Sit. Legs straight. Raise your arms. Lean back. Stretch upward.

2. Stretch forward and hold your ankles.

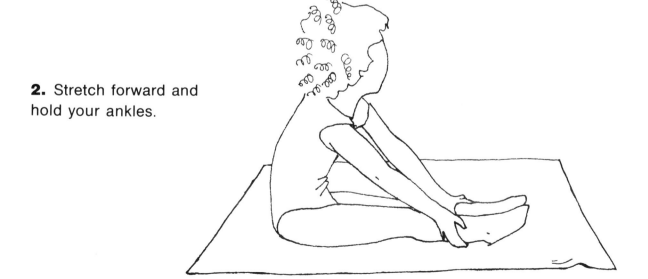

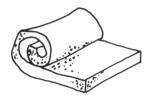

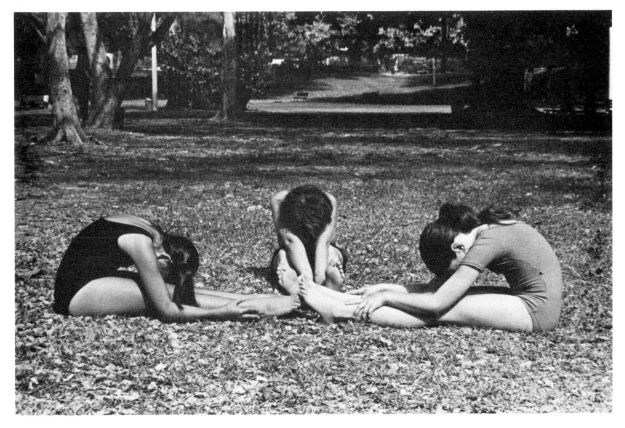

3. Bend your elbows and bring your forehead as close to your knees as you can. Try to touch your forehead to your knees. Hold. Count 10.

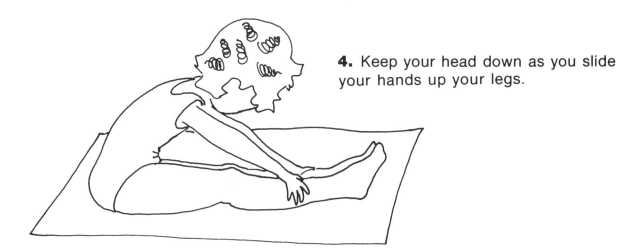

4. Keep your head down as you slide your hands up your legs.

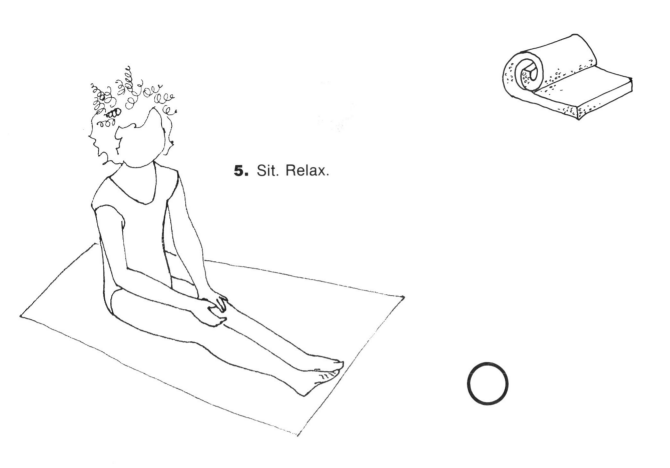

5. Sit. Relax.

HOW TO DO THE EXERCISE:

It may take a few weeks before you can get your head to touch your knees. Hold on to your legs and gently pull your forehead toward your legs. Do not pull hard or you will hurt yourself. If you cannot keep your knees straight at first, bend them slightly. After two weeks of counting 10, try for the count of 15. Count 15 for two weeks. Then try for the count of 20. Do the exercise twice.

WHAT THE EXERCISE DOES FOR YOU:

Keeps your back, legs, and neck loose

NOTE TO PARENTS AND TEACHERS:

The benefits are much like the ones in the Ballet Dancer exercise, but in this posture the stretch is mostly down the center of the back, while in the Ballet Dancer position, the stretch is more toward the sides of the back. Additional benefits to the children are: the circulation to the head and face is improved, the under-part of the legs is stretched, and the hip joints are kept flexible. Call the children's attention to the fact that the purpose of the hold position is to remain perfectly still. They are not to fidget. Remind them also to breathe naturally—never to hold their breath.

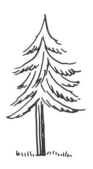

TREE

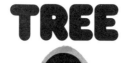

1. Place your right foot high up on the inside of your left thigh.

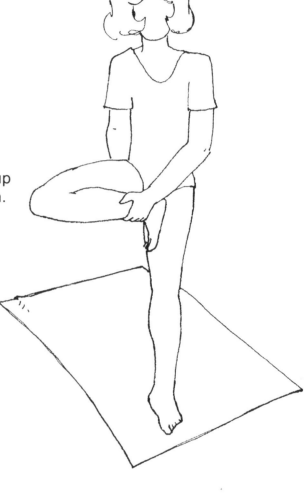

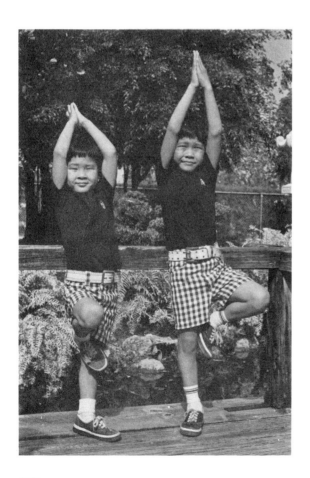

2. Raise your arms, palms touching. Hold. Count 5.

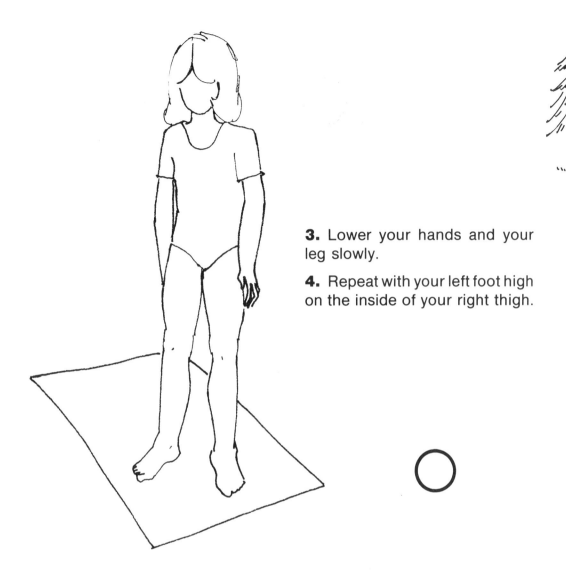

3. Lower your hands and your leg slowly.

4. Repeat with your left foot high on the inside of your right thigh.

HOW TO DO THE EXERCISE:

Try to bring your foot as high up on the inside of your thigh as you can.

After you have held the count of 5 for two weeks, try for the count of 10. Do not go past the count of 10. Do the exercise twice.

WHAT THE EXERCISE DOES FOR YOU:

Gives you better balance

NOTE TO PARENTS AND TEACHERS:

This exercise is fun to do and will soon have the children laughing. If they have difficulty balancing themselves at first, they can lean against the wall. Additional benefits are: the children improve their posture and their poise.

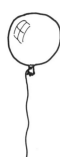

BALLOON

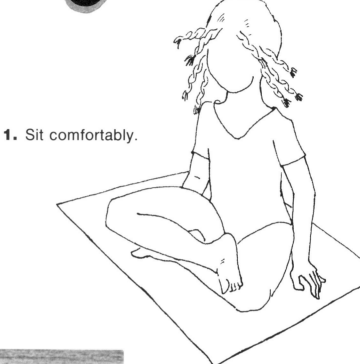

1. Sit comfortably.

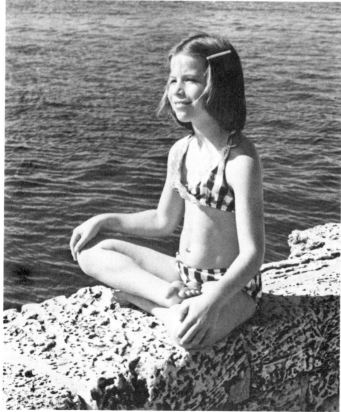

2. Breathe in and push your tummy out.

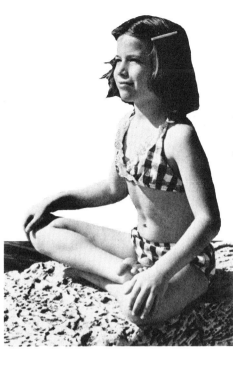

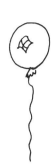

3. Continue to breathe in but pull your tummy in and push your chest out.

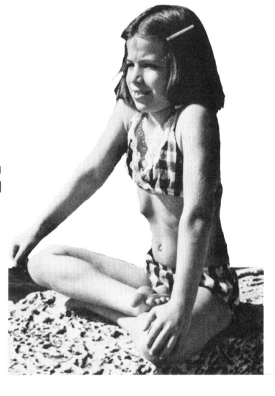

4. Breathe in further as you slowly raise your shoulders. Hold your breath for the count of 4.

5. Breathe out slowly through your nose. Lower your shoulders. Relax.

HOW TO DO THE EXERCISE:

It may take you one or two weeks before you learn to breathe in at the same time that you push your tummy out. Do steps 2, 3, and 4 with one long breath. Your movements must not be jerky. Read the directions many times to be sure that you are doing the exercise the right way. When you come out of the posture, just lower your shoulders and breathe out through your nose as much as you can.

After you have held the count of 4 for four weeks, add 2 counts every week until you can hold your breath for the count of 10. Do not go past the count of 10. Do the exercise 5 times.

WHAT THE EXERCISE DOES FOR YOU:

Brings more air into your lungs and makes your lungs strong

Relaxes you and helps you fall asleep

NOTE TO PARENTS AND TEACHERS:

When the Balloon exercise is done slowly and correctly, it is a marvelous relaxation technique. The slower the child breathes, the calmer he tends to become. He can do the exercise while sitting up in bed or at his desk in school. In bed, it induces him to fall easily into a peaceful sleep. At his desk in school, where he can do it many times during the day, it has a relaxing effect on him. The exercise will show results in two or three minutes.

Help the child to understand that the only way he can completely fill his lungs with air is to open them up from the bottom to the top. Pushing his belly out gives the lower part of his lungs the room to expand and fill with air. Pushing his chest out spreads his rib cage and gives the middle part of his lungs the room to expand. Raising his shoulders gives the upper portion of his lungs the room to expand.

Caution the child against attempting to hold his breath beyond the count of 10. Remind him that he is doing yoga exercises to keep himself healthy, and that he should not strain himself.

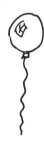

INTERMEDIATE EXERCISES

You have finished the beginning yoga exercises and are ready to go on to the exercises that are a little harder to do. They are called INTERMEDIATE exercises. Take two or three months to do them so that you learn them correctly. Be sure that you are ready for them before you begin.

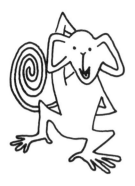

BACK SCRATC●

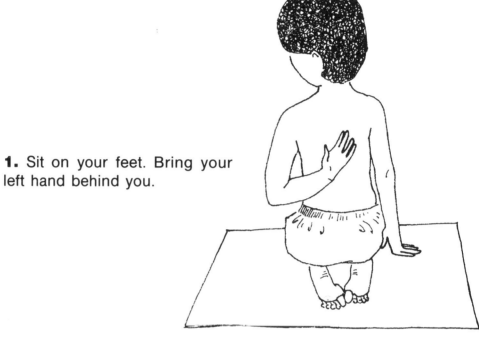

1. Sit on your feet. Bring your left hand behind you.

2. Reach over your shoulder with your right hand and put your fingers together. Hold. Count 5.

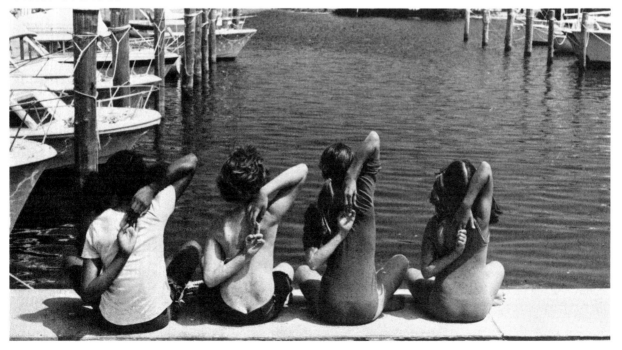

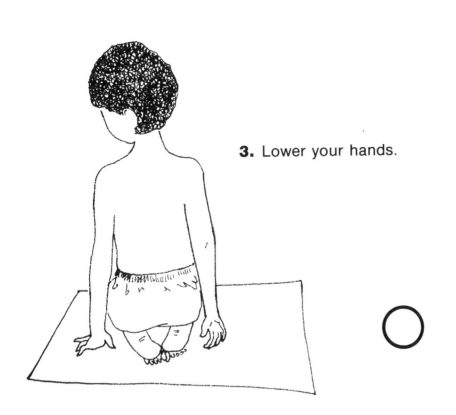

3. Lower your hands.

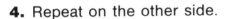

4. Repeat on the other side.

HOW TO DO THE EXERCISE:

It is not easy to get your fingers to touch. Practice a little every day so that you can get them to touch. If you are not comfortable kneeling, you may do the exercise with your legs crossed, sitting in the Tailor, the Lotus Bud, or the Lotus Flower position.

After you have held the count of 5 for two weeks, try for the count of 10. Do not go past the count of 10. Do the exercise twice.

WHAT THE EXERCISE DOES FOR YOU:

Helps you stand straight and tall

Keeps your arms, back, and shoulders from getting stiff

NOTE TO PARENTS AND TEACHERS:

This is a good exercise to do if the children have been sitting for a long time. It relieves fatigue in the shoulder areas and is invigorating.

CURLING LEAF

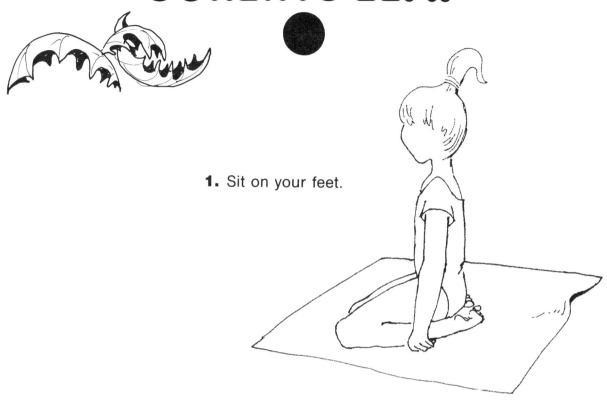

1. Sit on your feet.

2. Bend forward, placing your chest on your thighs, your forehead on the floor, your arms beside your legs. Hold. Count 10.

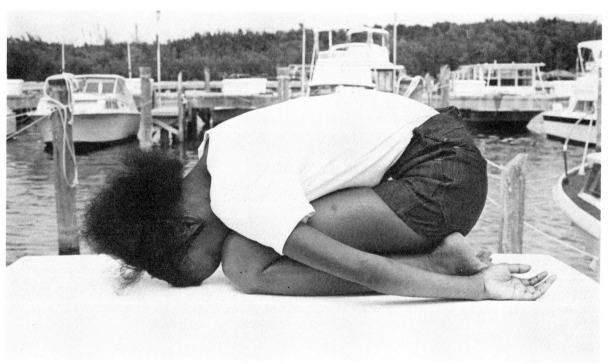

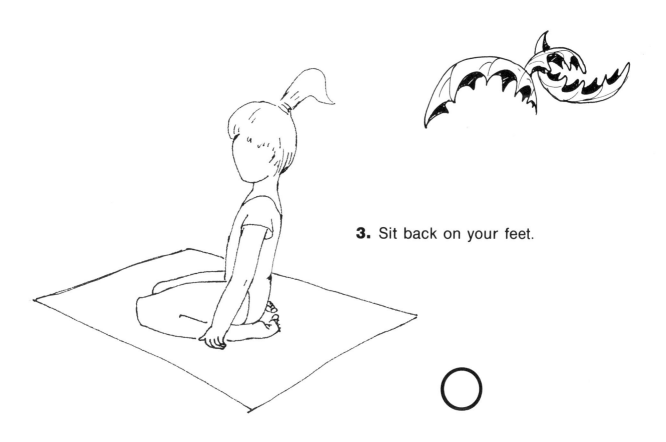

3. Sit back on your feet.

HOW TO DO THE EXERCISE:

Breathe slowly. Relax as much as you can. Keep your eyes closed the whole time you are doing this exercise.

Sit up slowly.

After you have held the count of 10 for two weeks, increase the count to 30. Hold the count of 30 for four weeks. Then try for the count of 60. Practice holding the count of 60 for four weeks. You may then hold the Curling Leaf posture for as long as you wish.

WHAT THE EXERCISE DOES FOR YOU:

Relaxes you and helps you sleep

NOTE TO PARENTS AND TEACHERS:

Once the child's legs and back have acquired the necessary flexibility, he will probably want to hold this posture often, as it is a naturally comfortable and relaxing position to assume.

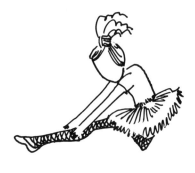

BALLET DANCER

●

1. Sit. Bring your left foot against your right thigh. Raise your arms. Lean back a little.

2. Hold your right ankle. Lower your head.

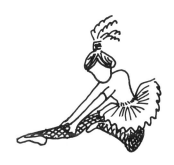

3. Bend your elbows. Bring your head down to your knee. Hold. Count 10.

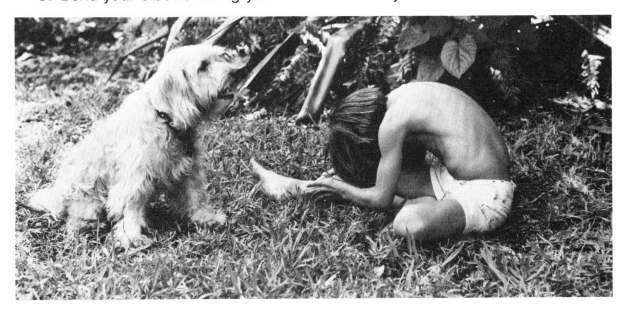

4. Keep your chin down. Slide your hands up your leg and slowly straighten up.

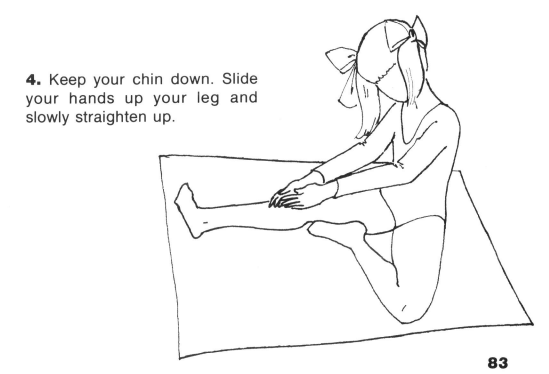

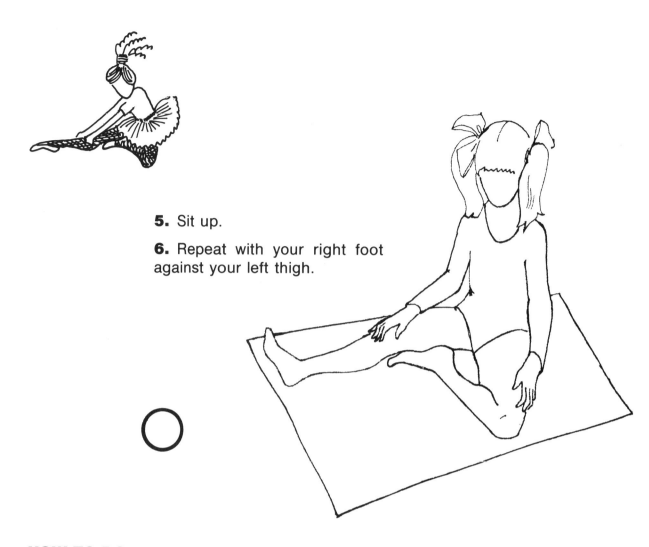

5. Sit up.

6. Repeat with your right foot against your left thigh.

HOW TO DO THE EXERCISE:

If you are not able to reach your ankle at first, hold on to the part of your leg you can reach. Try to get your forehead to touch your knee. Keeping your head down and your shoulders rounded when you are straightening up will let every bone in your spine feel the movement.

After two weeks of counting 10, try for the count of 15. Count 15 for four weeks. Then try for the count of 20. Do the exercise twice.

WHAT THE EXERCISE DOES FOR YOU:

Helps you stand straight and tall

NOTE TO PARENTS AND TEACHERS:

The Ballet Dancer, Plough, and Jelly Roll make up a complementary group of exercises and can be practiced as a series. All three exercises provide an excellent stretch for the neck, spine, and legs. They improve posture and circulation and eliminate tensions.

EAGLE SPREAD

1. Sit with your legs apart, hands on your knees.

2. Slide your hands slowly down your legs and hold your ankles.

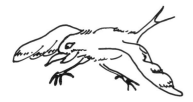

3. Pull yourself down. Bring your forehead to the floor. Hold. Count 5.

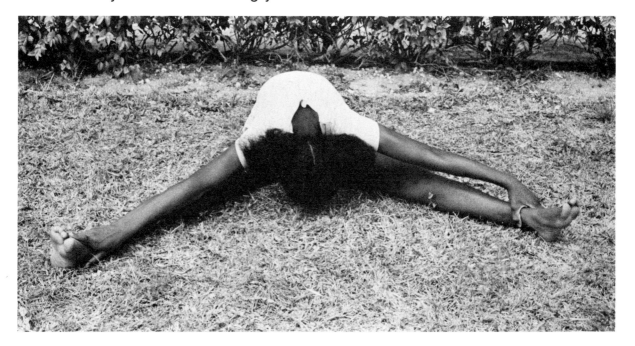

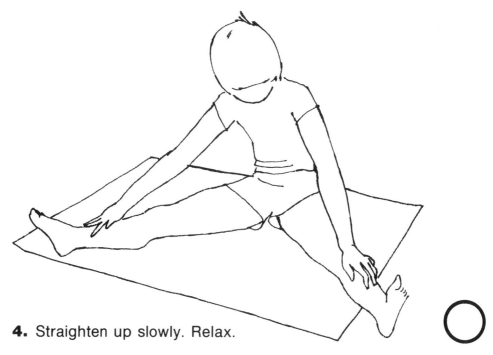

4. Straighten up slowly. Relax.

HOW TO DO THE EXERCISE:

Try to keep your legs as far apart as possible. Be careful not to pull too hard. After two weeks of counting 5, try for the count of 10. Count 10 for four weeks. Then try for the count of 20. Do the exercise twice.

WHAT THE EXERCISE DOES FOR YOU:

Helps your back to move and bend easily

Stretches your legs

NOTE TO PARENTS AND TEACHERS:

This exercise builds energy and improves the circulation of blood to the brain. It also keeps the spine limber and stretches the inside of the thighs. However, it is difficult to do. Caution the child to proceed slowly. Tell him his head will gradually move a little bit closer to the floor every week. In time, it will touch the floor.

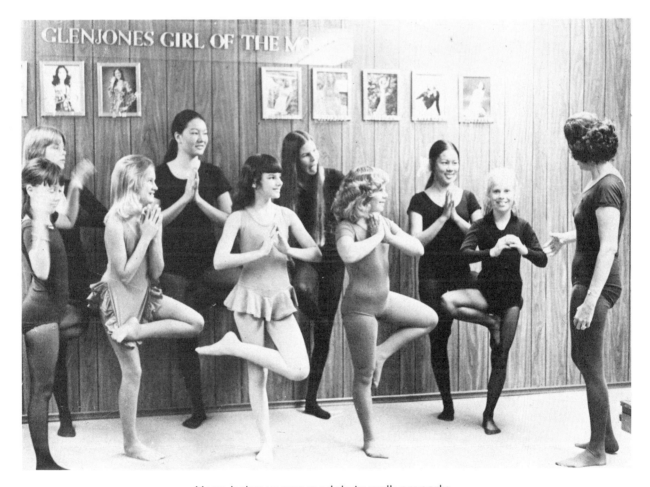

Yoga helps young models to walk properly.

HALF LOCUST

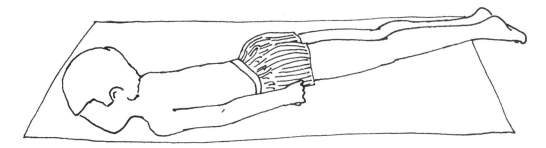

1. Lie on your tummy. Place your chin on the floor. Make fists with your hands. Keep your fists close to your body.

2. Press down with your chin and fists. Raise your right leg slowly. Hold. Count 5.

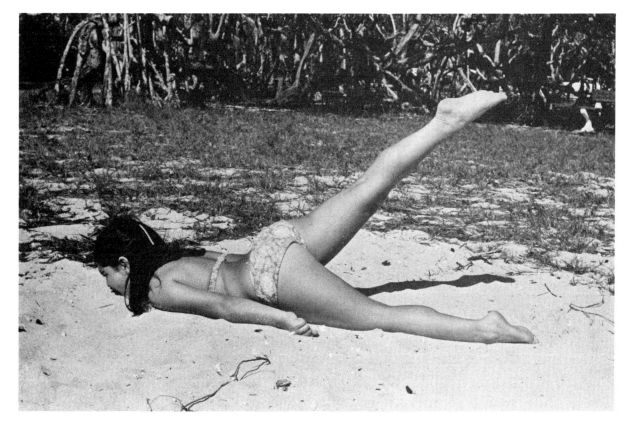

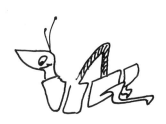

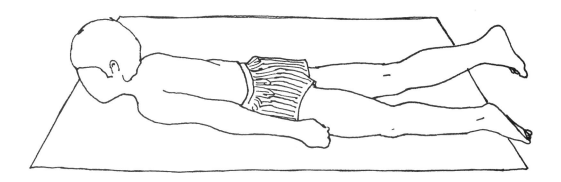

3. Lower your leg slowly.

4. Repeat with your other leg.

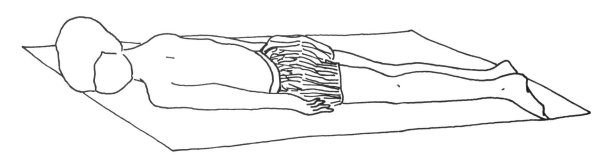

5. Rest with your cheek on the floor and your arms at your sides.

HOW TO DO THE EXERCISE:

Try to keep your leg straight. Do not shift your hips too much to the side when you raise a leg.

After you have held the count of 5 for four weeks, try for the count of 10. Do not go past the count of 10. Do the exercise twice.

WHAT THE EXERCISE DOES FOR YOU:

Strengthens your back

NOTE TO PARENTS AND TEACHERS:

This exercise is stimulating to the child because it increases the circulation to his head and face. The best time for him to practice it is in the afternoon or early evening.

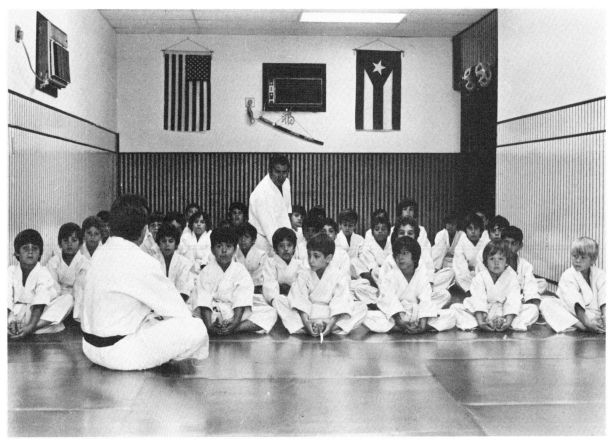

Here a Judo class sits in a yoga position.

RABBIT SIT

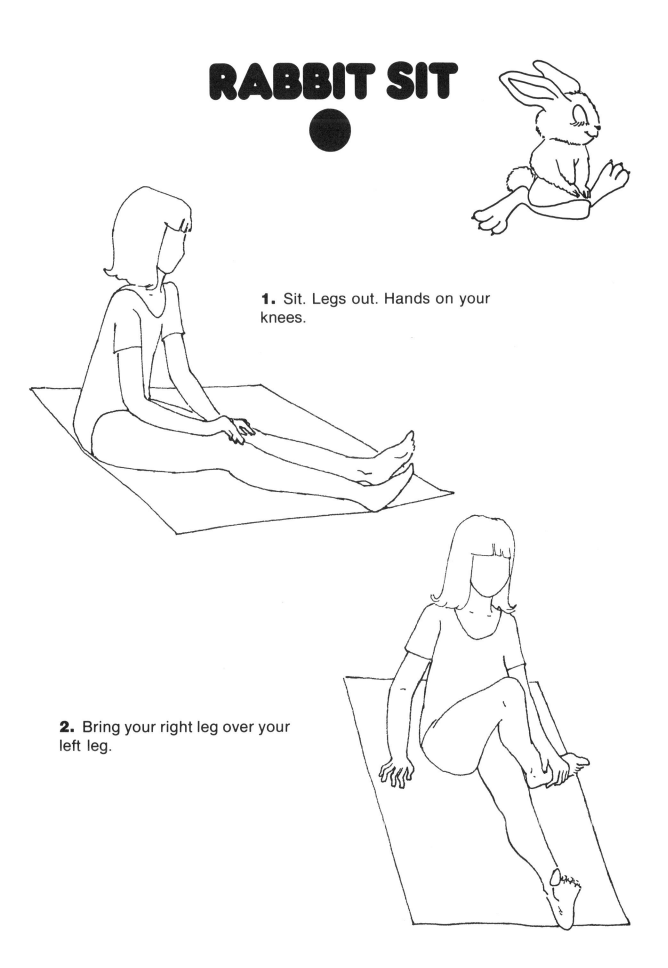

1. Sit. Legs out. Hands on your knees.

2. Bring your right leg over your left leg.

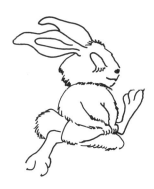

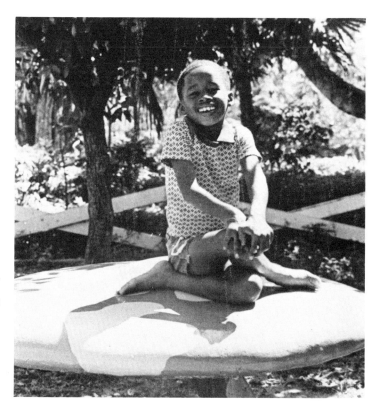

3. Bring your left foot under your right thigh. Place your hands on your knee. Hold. Count to 10.

4. Straighten your legs.

5. Repeat on the other side.

HOW TO DO THE EXERCISE:

Sit between your feet, not on your feet, and keep one knee over the other. Make sure that your back is straight, and that as you keep changing legs, first your right leg is on top, then your left leg. Change your legs often.

After you have held the count of 10 for two weeks, try for the count of 20. Count 20 for four weeks. Then try for the count of 30. When you reach 30, sit as long as you can comfortably. You can watch television or listen to the radio when you do the Rabbit Sit.

WHAT THE EXERCISE DOES FOR YOU:

Keeps your hips, knees, legs, and ankles loose

NOTE TO PARENTS AND TEACHERS:

This is a difficult technique. Even the small child lacks elasticity in his hip joints and in his legs. By practicing the Rabbit Sit and other hip and leg stretches, he can get the flexibility he needs. Flexibility in his hips and legs can give him an advantage in dancing, running, and any other sport he may undertake.

ROCKING
HORSE

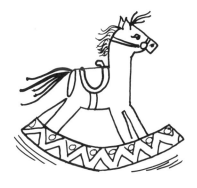

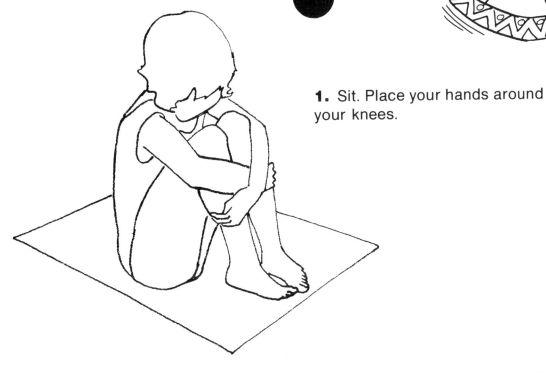

1. Sit. Place your hands around your knees.

2. Roll back and forth, keeping your knees close to your chest. Repeat 5 times.

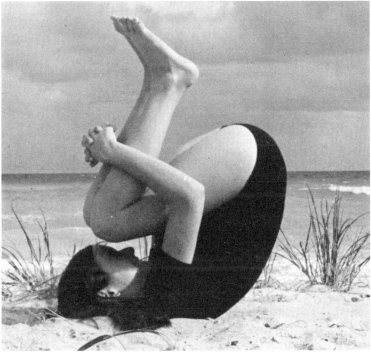

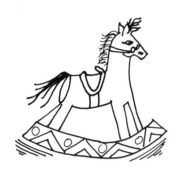

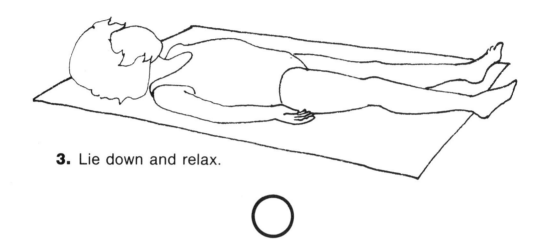

3. Lie down and relax.

HOW TO DO THE EXERCISE:

Be sure that you are lying on a rug or on a thick blanket. Do only 5 rolls and rest for the count of 5. You can do another 5 rolls after that.

WHAT THE EXERCISE DOES FOR YOU:

Warms your body and gives you energy

Massages your back

Makes you think better

NOTE TO PARENTS AND TEACHERS:

This is a fun exercise, stimulating and invigorating. The children will laugh as they perform it. They should not practice the exercise before bed, for they will not fall asleep.

TWINKLE TOES

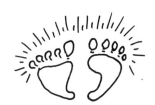

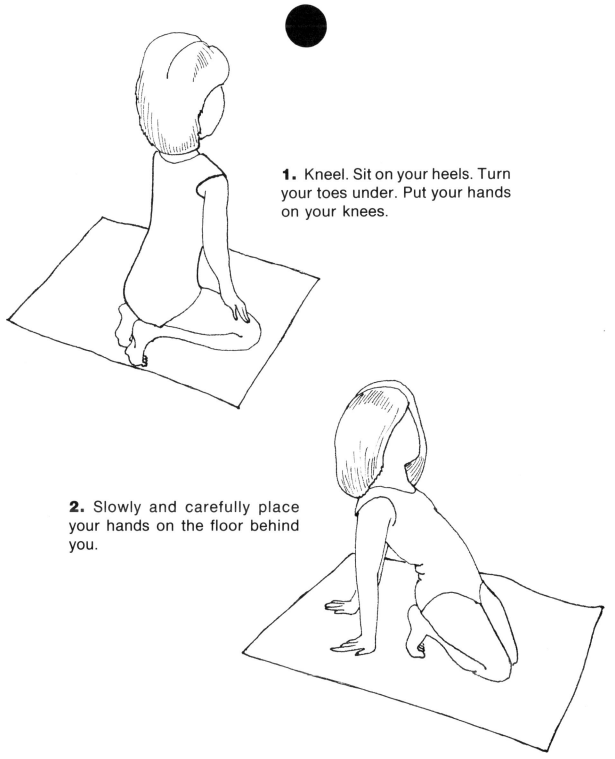

1. Kneel. Sit on your heels. Turn your toes under. Put your hands on your knees.

2. Slowly and carefully place your hands on the floor behind you.

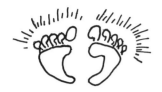

3. Drop your head back. Hold. Count 10.

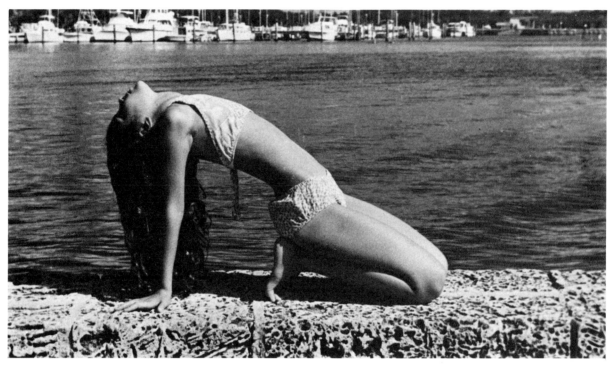

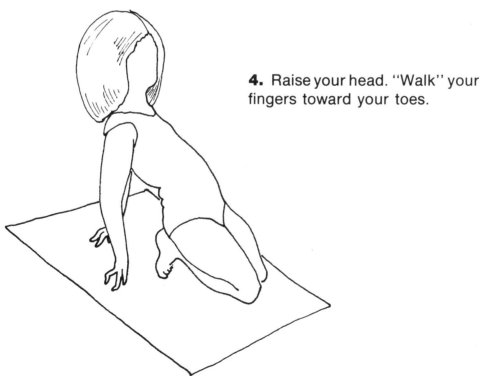

4. Raise your head. "Walk" your fingers toward your toes.

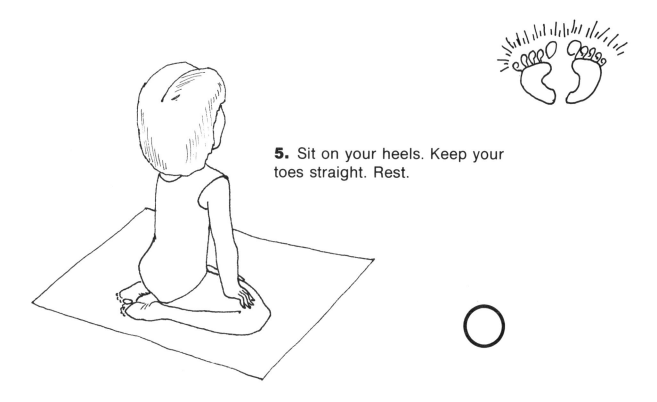

5. Sit on your heels. Keep your toes straight. Rest.

HOW TO DO THE EXERCISE:

You may be surprised to find that your toes are stiff and that you cannot sit easily on them. Do not be disturbed if it takes a few weeks before you can sit comfortably. You can practice sitting on your toes while watching television. Be sure that you do not bend back until it is easy for you to sit on them. Take your time learning the exercise. After you have held the count of 10 for two weeks, try for the count of 15. Count 15 for four weeks. Then try for the count of 20. Do the exercise twice.

WHAT THE EXERCISE DOES FOR YOU:

Strengthens your toes and makes them easy to move around

NOTE TO PARENTS AND TEACHERS:

Shoes do not allow the toes the leeway they need to bend, stretch, and grip. Since children wear shoes much of the time, their toes do not get all the free movement required. It is therefore important for the children to do this exercise often. They cannot, of course, wear shoes while performing it.

STAR

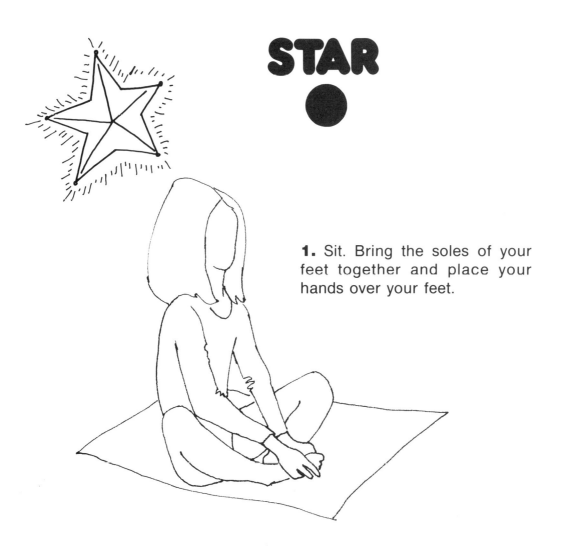

1. Sit. Bring the soles of your feet together and place your hands over your feet.

2. Slowly bend forward. Touch your forehead to your toes. Hold. Count 10.

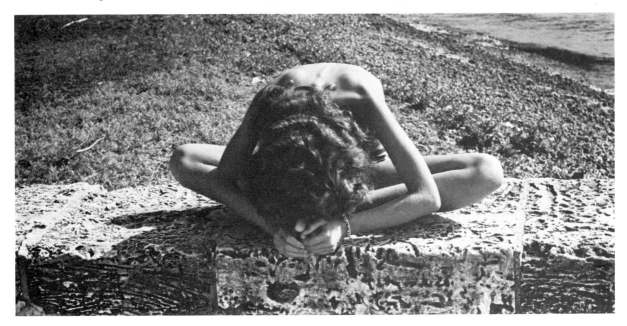

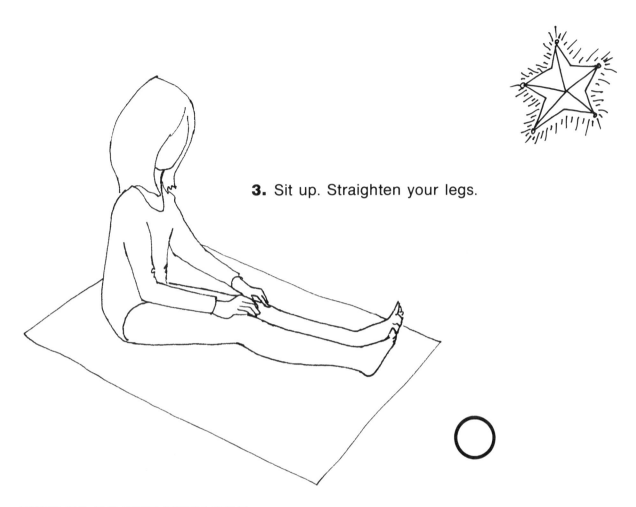

3. Sit up. Straighten your legs.

HOW TO DO THE EXERCISE:

It may take a few weeks before you are able to bring your forehead to your toes. Do not force your forehead to touch your toes. When you sit up, be sure you straighten your lower back first, then the middle of your back, then your neck. Raise your head last.

After you have held the count of 10 for two weeks, try for the count of 15. Count 15 for four weeks. Then try for the count of 20. Do the exercise twice.

WHAT THE EXERCISE DOES FOR YOU:

Stretches your legs and makes them easier for you to move

Keeps your back and neck loose

NOTE TO PARENTS AND TEACHERS:

This exercise and the Frog exercise are excellent for keeping the child's legs flexible. Ordinary walking and running do not stretch his legs sufficiently.

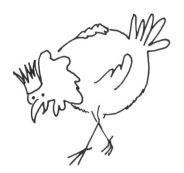

ROYAL HEN

●

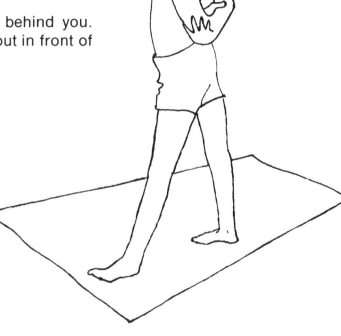

1. Fold your arms behind you. Bring your left leg out in front of you.

2. Bend forward. Lower your head. Try to bring your arms higher up on your back than they are. Hold. Count 5.

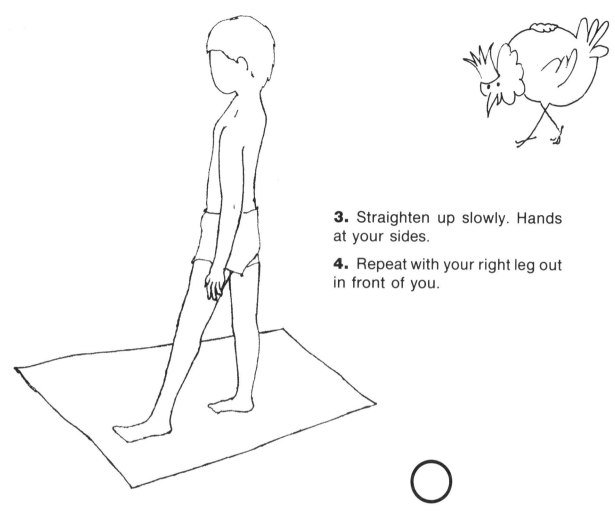

3. Straighten up slowly. Hands at your sides.

4. Repeat with your right leg out in front of you.

HOW TO DO THE EXERCISE:

Keep your eyes open and you will be better able to balance yourself.

After two weeks of counting 5, increase the count to 10. Do not go past the count of 10. Do the exercise twice.

WHAT THE EXERCISE DOES FOR YOU:

Gives you good posture

NOTE TO PARENTS AND TEACHERS:

The exercise eases a feeling of fatigue that develops in the back and shoulder areas after sitting or standing for a long while. It is an excellent stretch for the back, neck, and shoulders.

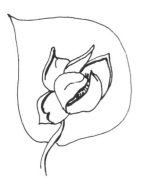

LOTUS BUD

●

1. Place your left foot against your right thigh.

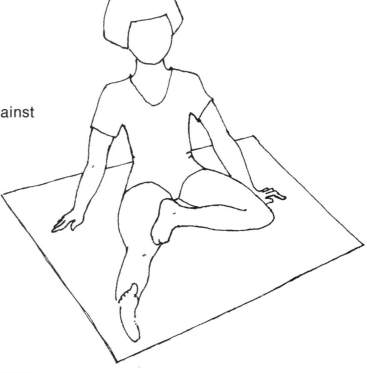

2. Bend your right leg and place it on top of your left leg. Hold. Count 30.

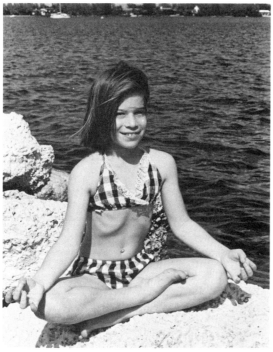

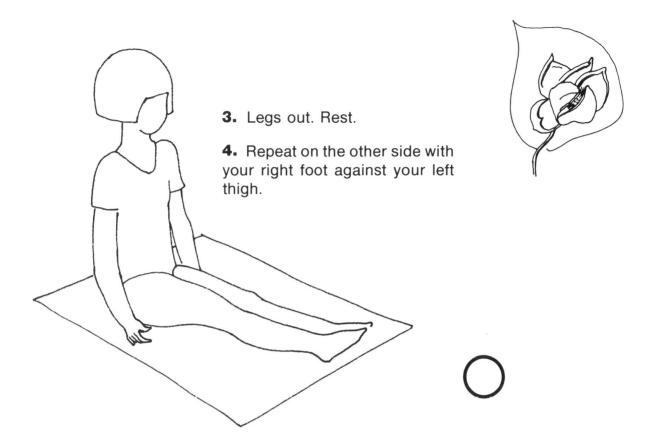

3. Legs out. Rest.

4. Repeat on the other side with your right foot against your left thigh.

HOW TO DO THE EXERCISE:

Keep changing sides. Try to keep your back straight. After two weeks of counting 30, add 10 every week until you reach 60. When you are sure your legs are comfortable, sit for as long as you like. This is a fun way to sit while watching television, while reading, or while talking to your friends.

WHAT THE EXERCISE DOES FOR YOU:

Keeps your legs from getting stiff

NOTE TO PARENTS AND TEACHERS:

This exercise not only benefits the child's legs; it regulates his breathing and soothes his mind.

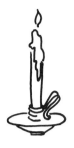

CANDLE

●

1. Lie on your back. Turn your palms down. Slowly raise your legs.

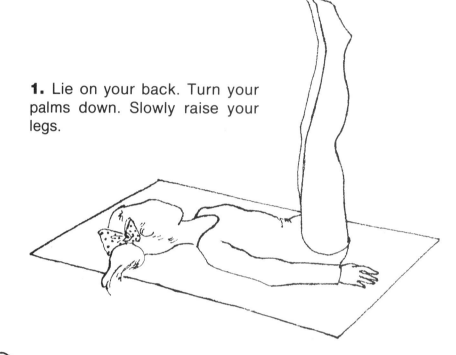

2. Push your hands down hard against the floor and raise your hips.

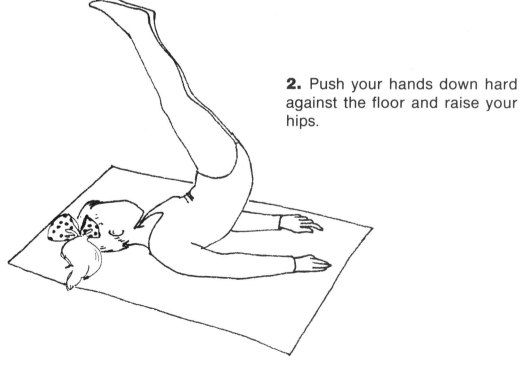

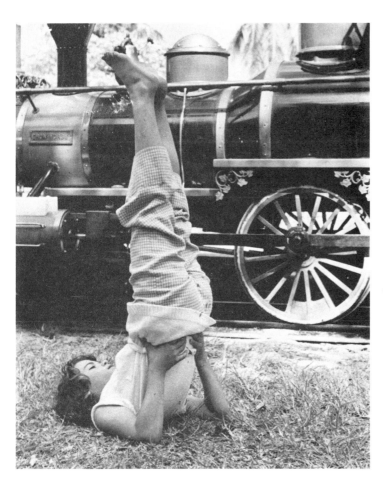

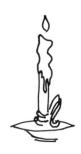

3. Place your hands against your back. Hold. Count to 30.

4. Slowly lower your knees to your forehead.

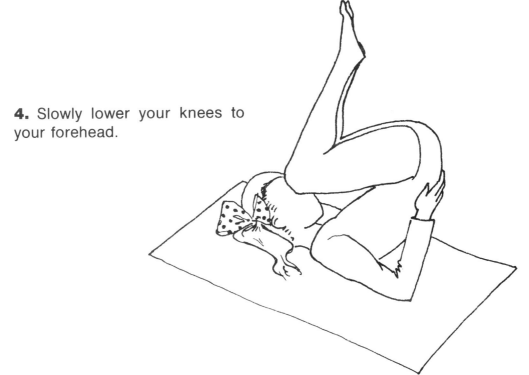

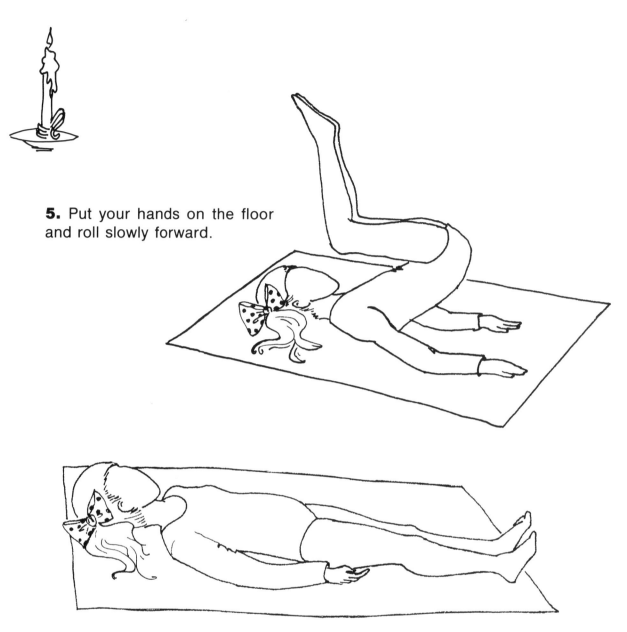

5. Put your hands on the floor and roll slowly forward.

6. Rest. Let yourself get limp all over. Turn your palms up.

HOW TO DO THE EXERCISE:

Be sure that your head, neck, and back are resting on a soft cover. Keep your chin in the middle of your chest. Try to keep your body straight when your legs are in the air. Count to 30 for one week. Then add 10 every week until you get to 60. Stop at 60 for two weeks. Then add 10 again every week. When you reach the count of 120 (2 minutes), do not go any further. Do this exercise once every day.

WHAT THE EXERCISE DOES FOR YOU:

Keeps you from getting too fat or too thin

Makes your tummy firm and your back strong

Rests your legs

NOTE TO PARENTS AND TEACHERS:

This exercise is excellent for children who have poor circulation in their legs. It also aids in controlling their weight. When the body is inverted, there is increased circulation to the throat area. This nourishes the thyroid gland, which plays a part in controlling weight. The best time for a child to do the Candle is in the late afternoon or evening.

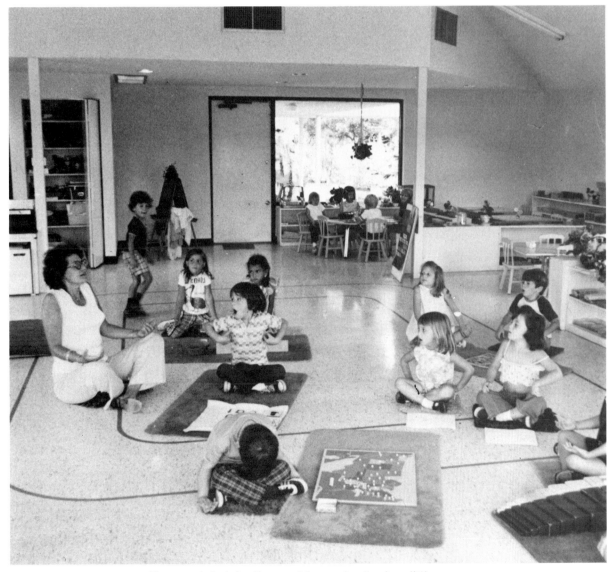

Nursery tots take time out from play to do a little yoga.

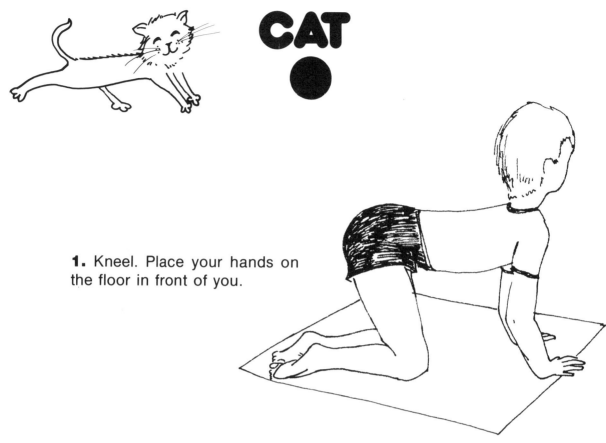

CAT

1. Kneel. Place your hands on the floor in front of you.

2. Bring your right knee to your forehead. Hold. Count 5.

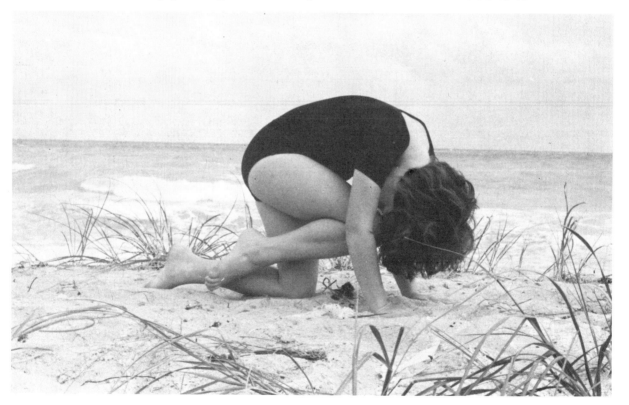

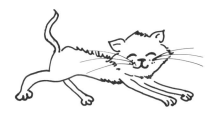

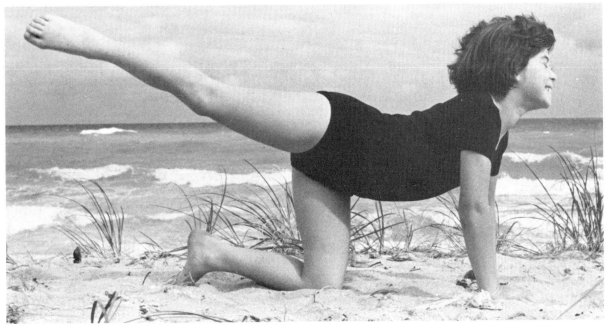

3. Raise and stretch your right leg back. Raise your head. Hold. Count 5.

4. Kneel and sit back on your heels. Rest.

5. Repeat with your left leg.

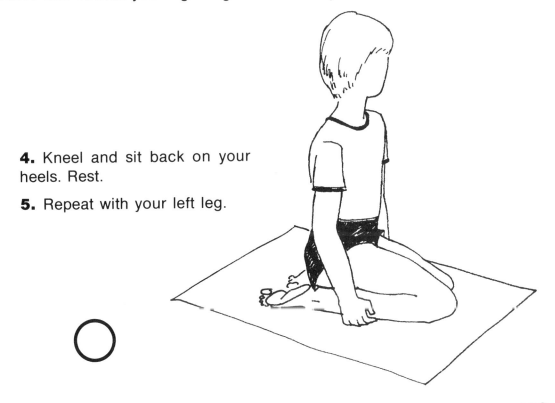

HOW TO DO THE EXERCISE:

When you bring your knee to your forehead, be sure that your foot does not touch the ground. Try not to bend your knee or move your hips as you raise your leg.

After you have held the count of 5 for two weeks, try for the count of 10. Do not go past the count of 10. Do the exercise twice.

WHAT THE EXERCISE DOES FOR YOU:

Keeps your back loose so you can move around easily

NOTE TO PARENTS AND TEACHERS:

Suggest that the children purr like a cat as they move gracefully and very catlike from stretch to stretch.

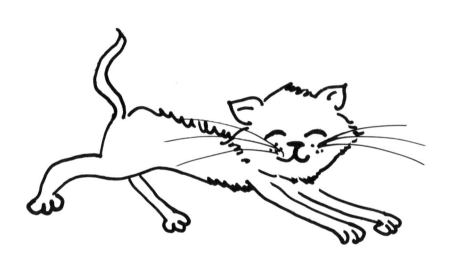

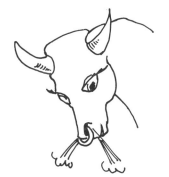

SNORTING BULL

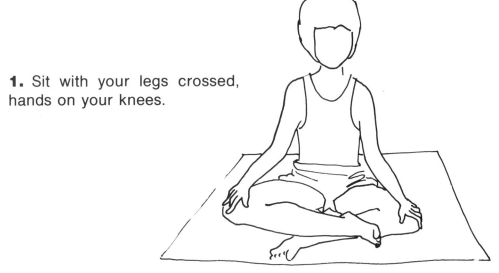

1. Sit with your legs crossed, hands on your knees.

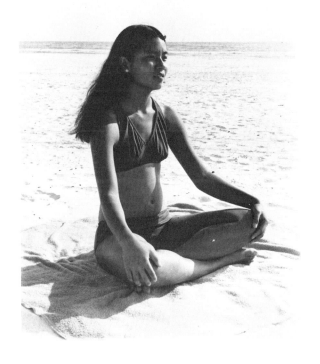

2. Slowly breathe in through your nose at the same time that you push your tummy out.

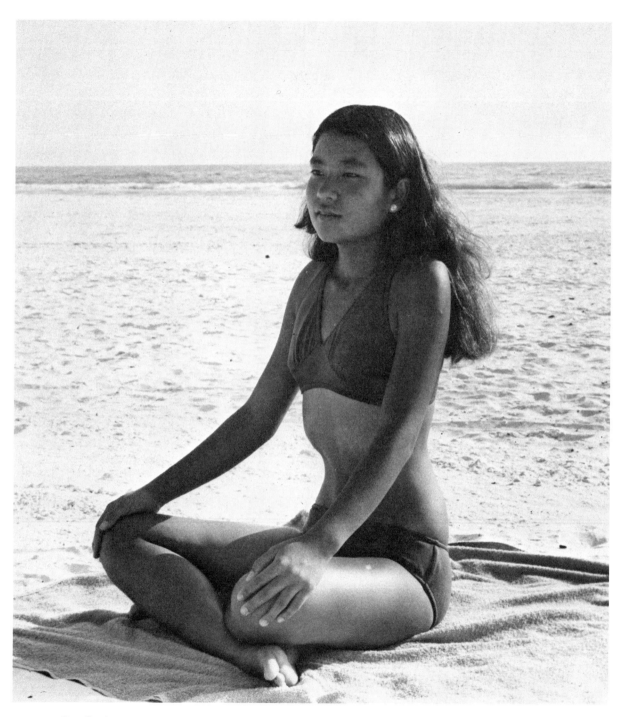

3. Quickly breathe out through your nose as you pull your tummy in.

4. Relax.

HOW TO DO THE EXERCISE:

Notice that you must breathe in slowly through your nose and breathe out quickly through your nose. Breathe in to the count of 3 and breathe out to the count of 1. Do this exercise 10 times. Rest. Do it 10 times again. Rest.

WHAT THE EXERCISE DOES FOR YOU:

Brings air quickly into your lungs

Keeps your nose and lungs clean

Warms your body

Helps you to think better

NOTE TO PARENTS AND TEACHERS:

This exercise has special benefits in that it clears the lungs of accumulated mucus. Even a very young child, who has not yet learned how to blow his nose, can use this technique.

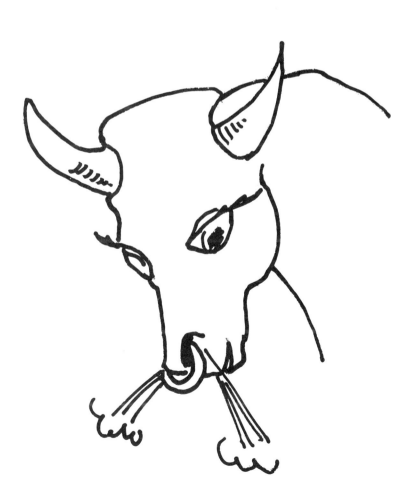

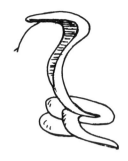

COBRA

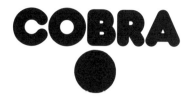

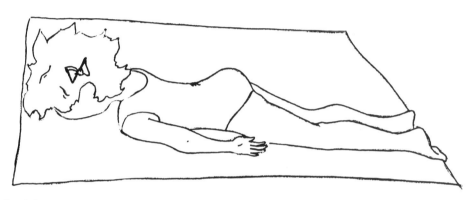

1. Lie on your tummy, hands at your sides. Place your forehead on the floor.

2. Raise your head.

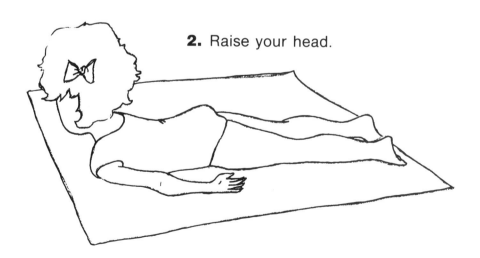

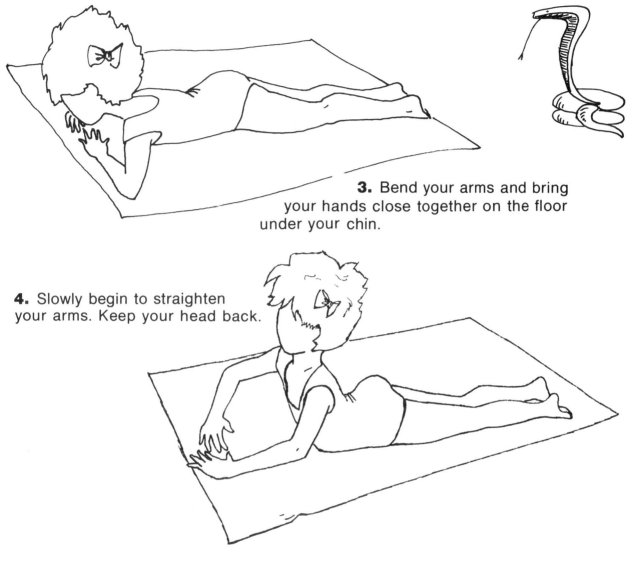

3. Bend your arms and bring your hands close together on the floor under your chin.

4. Slowly begin to straighten your arms. Keep your head back.

5. When your arms are straight, hold. Count 10.

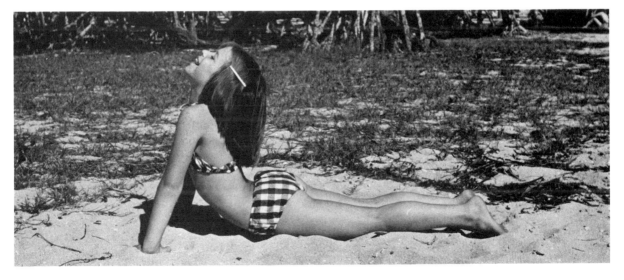

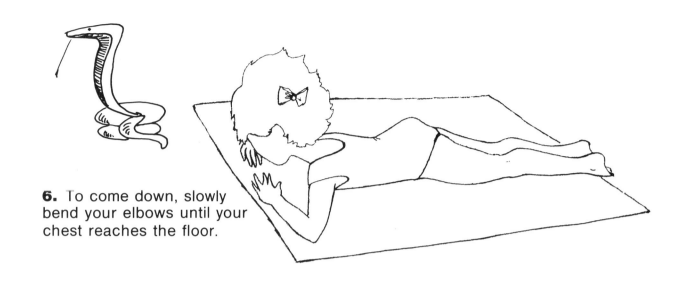

6. To come down, slowly bend your elbows until your chest reaches the floor.

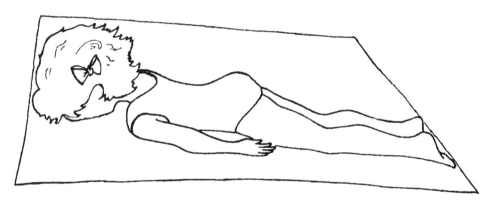

7. Bring your hands to your sides. Place your forehead on the floor.

8. Turn your head to the side. Rest.

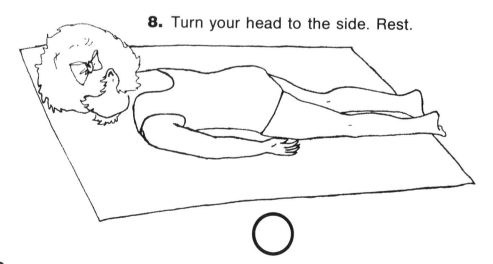

HOW TO DO THE EXERCISE:

Be sure that you move slowly in every step of the Cobra exercise. As you come down, your tummy will touch the floor first, then your chest, then your chin. Your forehead should touch last. See if you can hiss like a snake.

After you have held the count of 10 for two weeks, try for the count of 15. Count 15 for four weeks. Then try for the count of 20. Do not go past the count of 20. Do the exercise twice.

WHAT THE EXERCISE DOES FOR YOU:

Increases your energy

Keeps your back and neck loose

NOTE TO PARENTS AND TEACHERS:

The child can adjust the position of his arms to suit his body. If his back is very stiff, instead of placing his hands directly under his chin, let him place his hands farther out in front of his face. As his back becomes more limber, he can bring his hands closer in toward his chin. If he pretends that he is a snake slithering in and out of this exercise, his movements will not be jerky or rushed.

Although the Cobra technique increases the child's energy through improved circulation, it also relaxes him because it relieves tension. Even if the child has only a few minutes available, it is a good exercise to do because it brings relaxation quickly.

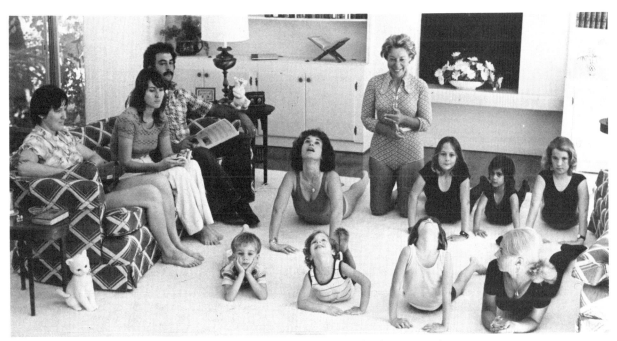

Sometimes, mommies and daddies join the yoga classes.

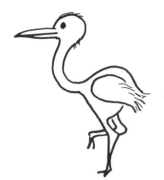

STORK

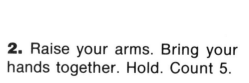

1. Stand on your left leg and place your right foot high on your left thigh.

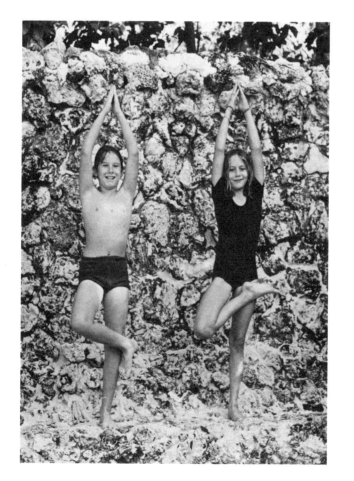

2. Raise your arms. Bring your hands together. Hold. Count 5.

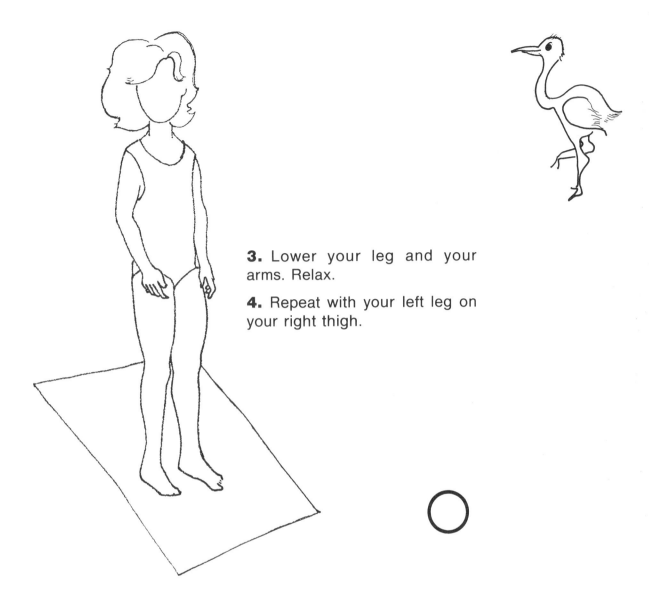

3. Lower your leg and your arms. Relax.

4. Repeat with your left leg on your right thigh.

HOW TO DO THE EXERCISE:

To keep your balance, look at an object straight ahead of you that is not moving.

After you have held the count of 5 for two weeks, try for the count of 10. Do not go past the count of 10. Do the exercise twice.

WHAT THE EXERCISE DOES FOR YOU:

Helps you to fix your mind on what you are doing

Improves your balance

NOTE TO PARENTS AND TEACHERS:

Improved balance helps children move gracefully. This is a fun exercise. There will be much giggling as they attempt to keep from falling over.

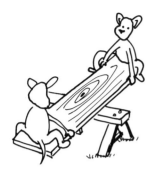

SEESAW

1. Sit with your hands on the floor beside you. Raise your legs. Balance yourself.

2. Touch your right ankle with your right hand. Balance yourself.

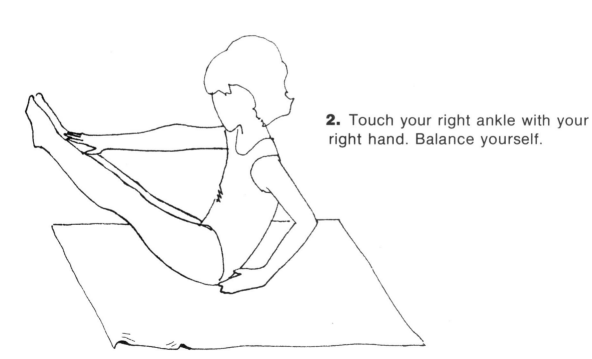

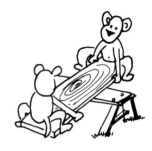

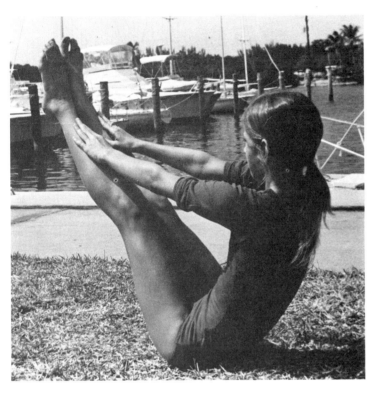

3. Touch both ankles. Balance yourself. Hold. Count 5.

4. Legs down. Rest.

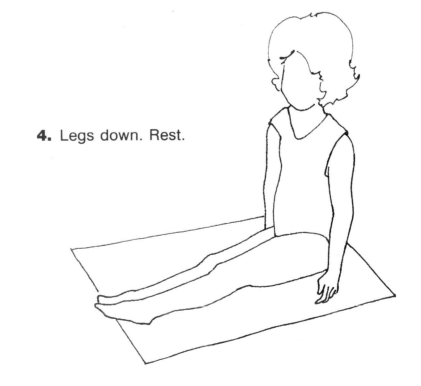

HOW TO DO THE EXERCISE:

Do this exercise on a padded floor. After you have held the count of 5 for two weeks, try for the count of 10. Do not go past the count of 10. Do the exercise twice.

WHAT THE EXERCISE DOES FOR YOU:

Gives you better balance

Strengthens your back and tummy muscles

Helps you to keep your mind on whatever you do

NOTE TO PARENTS AND TEACHERS:

Fun and good health go together in yoga. While the child is having fun doing this deceptively simple exercise, he is also developing his strength and stamina.

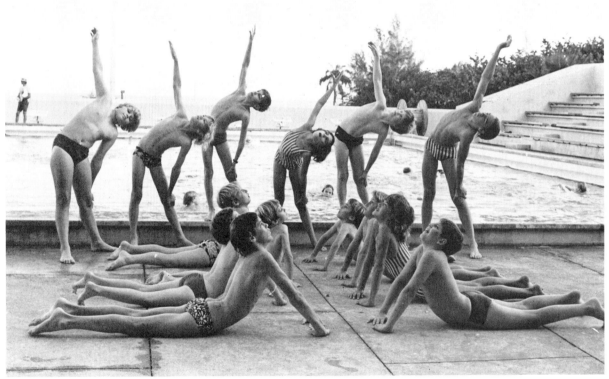

This swimming team keeps in shape with yoga.

SLIDE

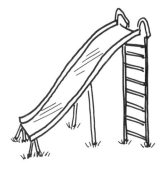

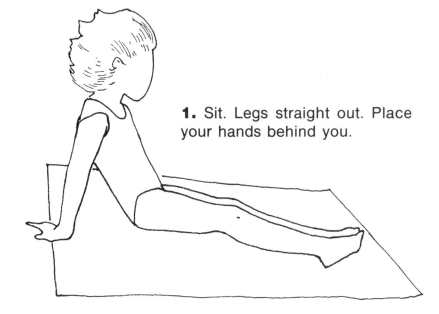

1. Sit. Legs straight out. Place your hands behind you.

2. Push your hands down hard. Push your back up. Drop your head back. Hold. Count 5.

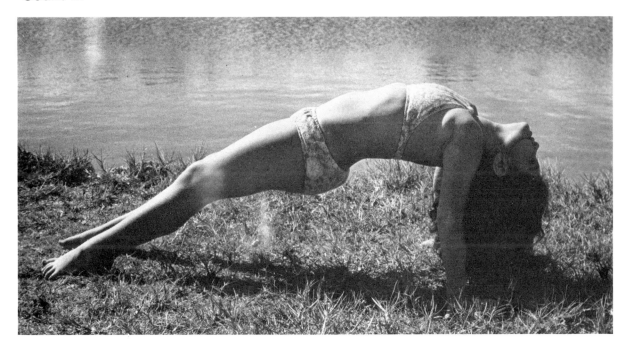

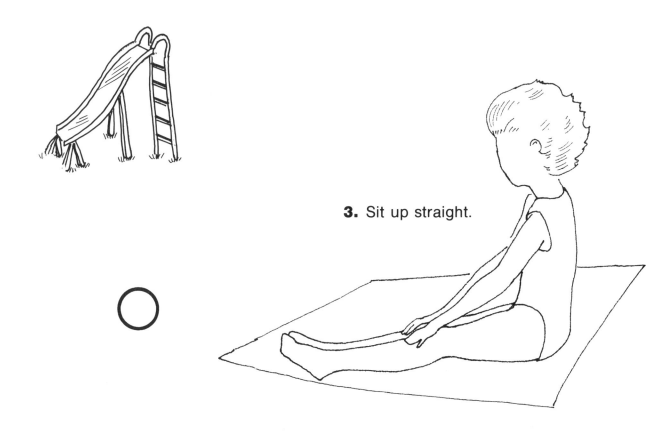

3. Sit up straight.

HOW TO DO THE EXERCISE:

Be sure your toes touch the floor when you hold the exercise. Let your head drop back all the way. Try to keep your knees straight. Since your arms do all the work in pushing, you will have to push hard to get up.

After you have held the count of 5 for two weeks, try for the count of 10. Do not go past the count of 10. Do the exercise twice.

WHAT THE EXERCISE DOES FOR YOU:

Makes your arms and shoulders strong

NOTE TO PARENTS AND TEACHERS:

This exercise is harder than it looks. If a child has too little strength in his arms, it will be difficult for him to get his toes to touch the floor. It should only take a week or two, however, to increase the strength in his arms. The Slide technique keeps the child's neck and back flexible and brings increased circulation to his head, face, and scalp.

ADVANCED EXERCISES

Now you have come to the ADVANCED yoga exercises, and some of them are very difficult to do. Practice only two or three new ones each week. Take your time learning them, and remember, never *force* yourself to do an exercise you are not ready to do.

FLY AWAY BIRD

●

1. Stand with your hands at your sides.

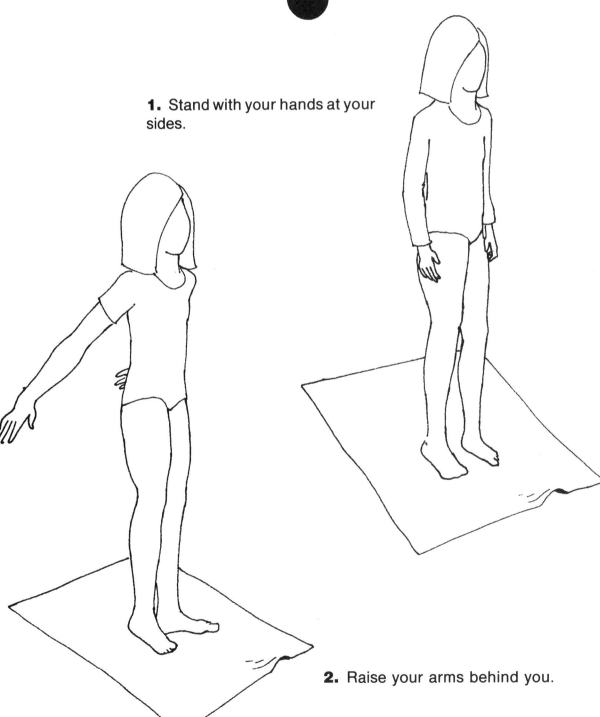

2. Raise your arms behind you.

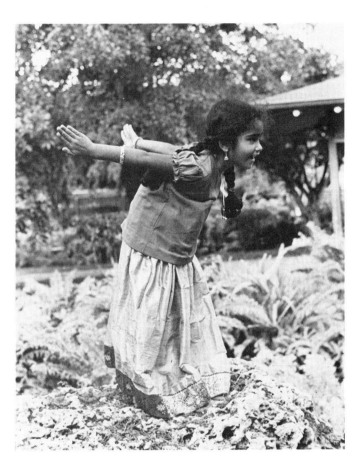

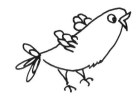

3. Rise up high on your toes and lean forward a little. Hold. Count 5.

4. Bring your heels back to the floor. Hands at your sides.

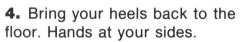

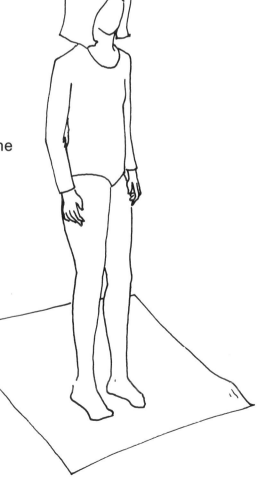

HOW TO DO THE EXERCISE:

Do not lean too far forward, or you will lose your balance.

After you have held the count of 5 for two weeks, try for the count of 10. Do not go past the count of 10. Do the exercise twice.

WHAT THE EXERCISE DOES FOR YOU:

Gives you better balance and helps you dance and walk gracefully

NOTE TO PARENTS AND TEACHERS:

Like all balancing techniques, this one is a little difficult at first. Do not expect the child to balance himself immediately. However, he should acquire some skill in a reasonably short period of time.

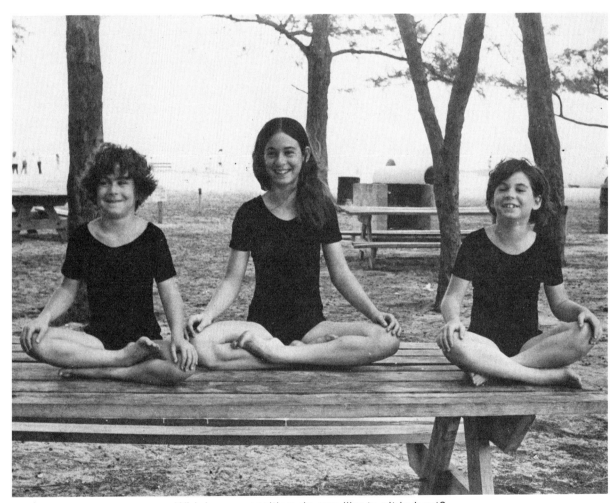

Which yoga position do you like to sit in best?

LOTUS FLOWER

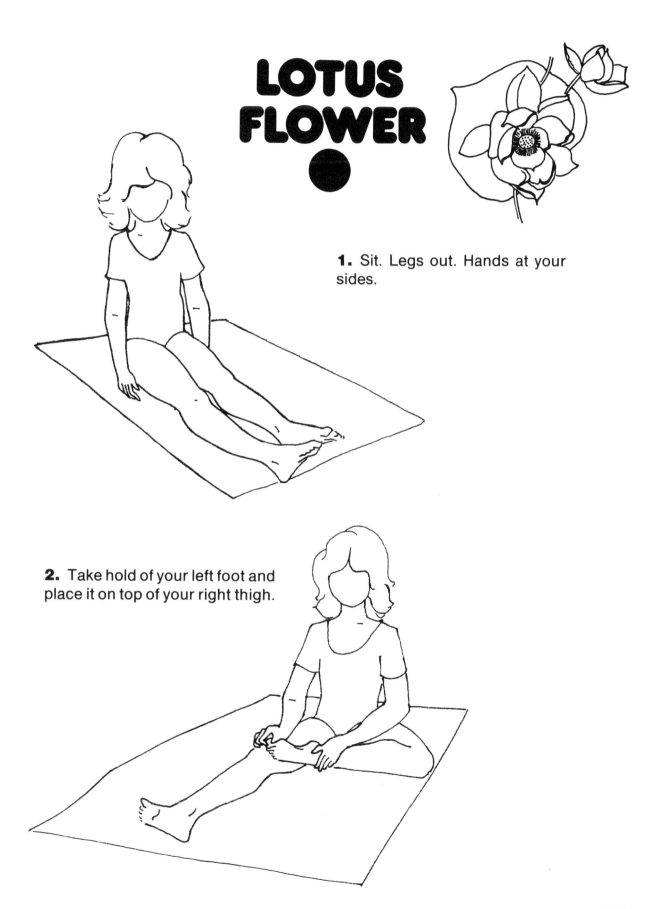

1. Sit. Legs out. Hands at your sides.

2. Take hold of your left foot and place it on top of your right thigh.

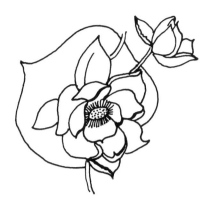

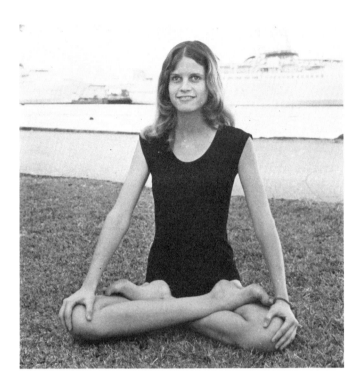

3. Take hold of your right foot and place it on top of your left thigh. Hands on your knees. Hold. Count 10.

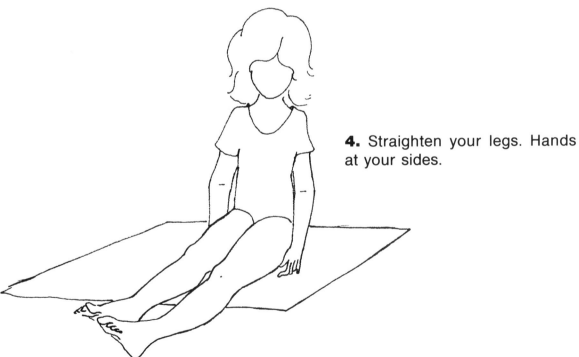

4. Straighten your legs. Hands at your sides.

5. Now do the exercise starting with your right foot. Put your right foot on top of your left thigh. Then put your left foot on top of your right thigh.

When you are in the Lotus Flower position and feel that you can do the exercise easily, try to push your hands down hard against the floor and raise your legs off the floor. It should be fun to see how high you can raise yourself from the floor. Look at the girl in the picture.

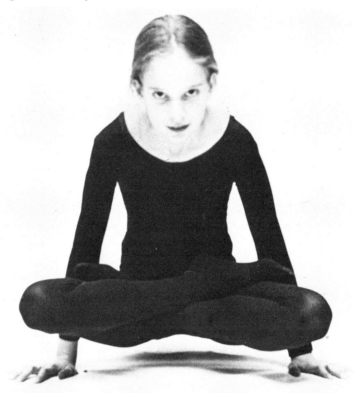

HOW TO DO THE EXERCISE:

Never push or pull your legs to get into this position. Continue changing your legs.

Sit for the count of 10 for two weeks. Then try for the count of 20. Sit for the count of 20 for two weeks. Then try for the count of 30. Sit for the count of 30 for two weeks. Then add 10 each week until you reach the count of 60. When you are sure that your legs are comfortable, sit as long as you can. You can read, write, or watch television while you practice the Lotus Flower position.

WHAT THE EXERCISE DOES FOR YOU:

Gives you strong, healthy legs so that you can move around easily

NOTE TO PARENTS AND TEACHERS:

Caution the child not to force his legs into the Lotus Flower position. If his legs are not ready to stretch into this advanced sitting posture, guide him instead into sitting in the Lotus Bud posture for a few weeks longer. It takes time for the child's ankles, knees, and hip joints to acquire the necessary flexibility to do this exercise.

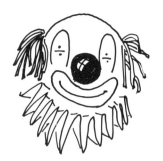

NOSEY CLOWN

●

1. Sit comfortably.

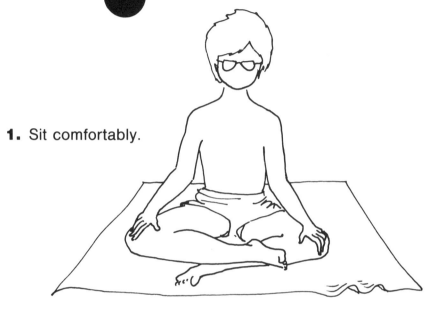

2. Press your right thumb gently against the right side of your nose. Place your first and second fingers between your eyebrows. Keep your third and little fingers together above the left side of your nose. The left side of your nose is open. Breathe in slowly through the left side of your nose.

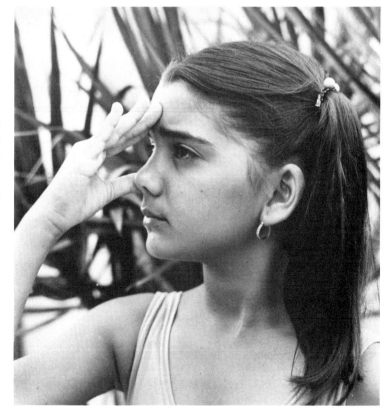

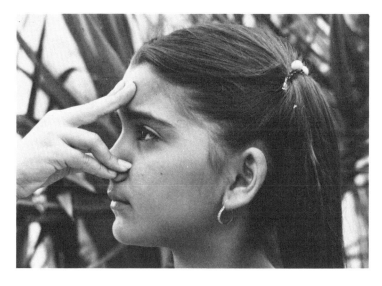

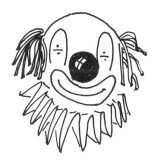

3. Close both sides of your nose and hold your breath.

4. Raise your thumb and breathe out slowly through the right side of your nose.

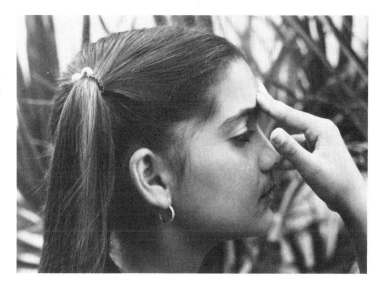

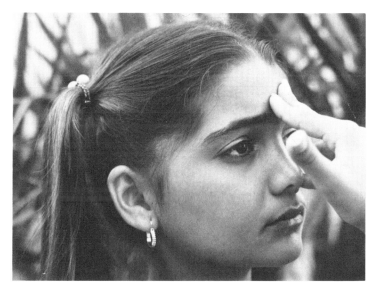

5. Breathe in slowly through the right side of your nose.

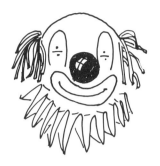

6. Close both sides of your nose. Hold your breath.

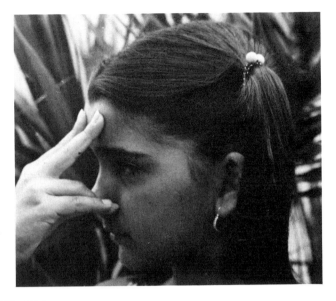

7. Raise your fourth and fifth fingers (pinky and the one next to it) and breathe out slowly through the left side of your nose.

8. You have now done the Nosey Clown breathing exercise for one round.

Let us review the steps:

Breathe in through the left side of your nose.

Hold your breath.

Breathe out through the right side of your nose.

Breathe in through the right side of your nose.

Hold your breath.

Breathe out through the left side of your nose.

This is one round.

HOW TO DO THE EXERCISE:

Be sure that you breathe in and out slowly. Count 4 as you breathe in, count 4 as you hold your breath, and count 4 as you breathe out. Do not count aloud. Do four rounds.

After two weeks of counting 4, increase the count to 6. Count 6 to breathe in, count 6 to hold your breath, and count 6 to breathe out. Do six rounds.

After two more weeks, count 8 to breathe in, count 8 to hold your breath, and count 8 to breathe out. Do eight rounds. Do not go past the count of 8.

WHAT THE EXERCISE DOES FOR YOU:

Helps you calm down and fall asleep

NOTE TO PARENTS AND TEACHERS:

When a child becomes edgy, he tends to breathe quickly and erratically. You can teach him how to slow down the rate at which he inhales and exhales. You can use the Nosey Clown exercise to relax him. It works in two or three minutes and can be done at any time. If done while sitting in bed, it will bring on sleep in moments. Just tell the child to close his eyes and concentrate on his breathing.

Actually, this is a complicated technique and may be difficult for very small children to learn. For them, substitute the Balloon exercise, which also uses a slow rate of breathing as a calming technique.

Yoga exercises help you fall asleep.

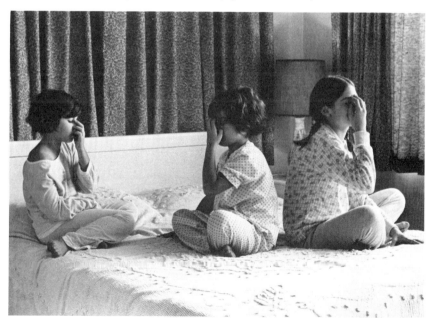

The Nosey Clown is a **good** exercise to do before going to bed.

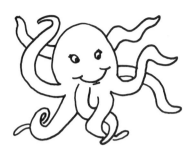

OCTOPUS

●

1. Stand. Place your left elbow inside your right elbow. Your hands and fingers should touch.

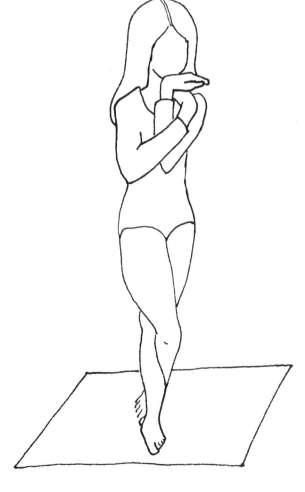

2. Swing your right leg over your left leg and tuck your right foot behind your left ankle. Place your chin on your hands.

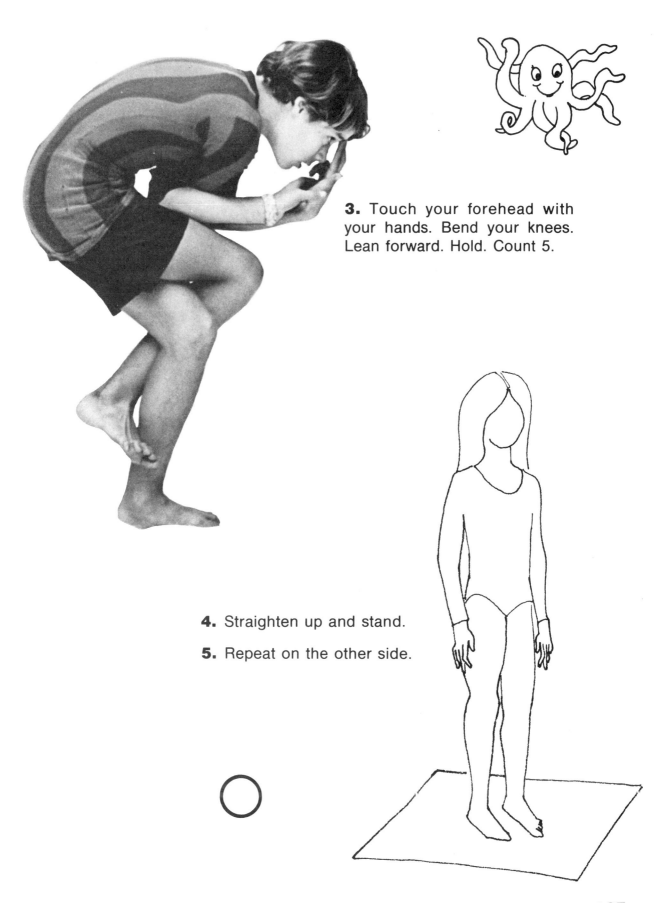

3. Touch your forehead with your hands. Bend your knees. Lean forward. Hold. Count 5.

4. Straighten up and stand.

5. Repeat on the other side.

HOW TO DO THE EXERCISE:

Make sure that you can balance yourself before you bend your knees and lean forward.

After you have held the count of 5 for two weeks, try for the count of 10. Do not go past the count of 10. Do the exercise twice.

WHAT THE EXERCISE DOES FOR YOU:

Helps your legs to move freely

Teaches you to balance yourself

Teaches you to pay attention to what you are doing

NOTE TO PARENTS AND TEACHERS:

It may take a few weeks of practice before the child can tuck his foot behind his ankle, and many more weeks before he can balance well enough to bend his knees. Caution him to do the exercise on a soft surface at first in case he should fall over.

This is a good exercise for the child to do after he has been sitting for a long time. While providing him with desirable movement, it can also bring him some fun and laughter.

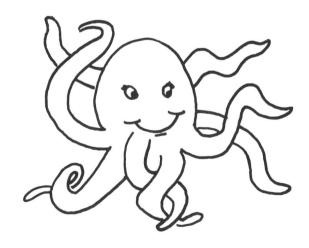

PYRAMID

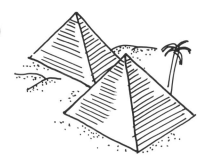

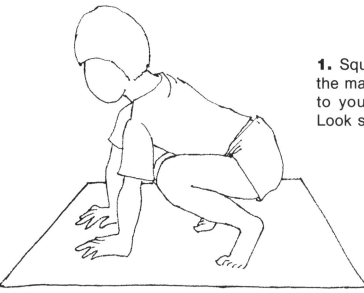

1. Squat. Place your hands on the mat. Keep your knees close to your chest, your heels up. Look straight ahead.

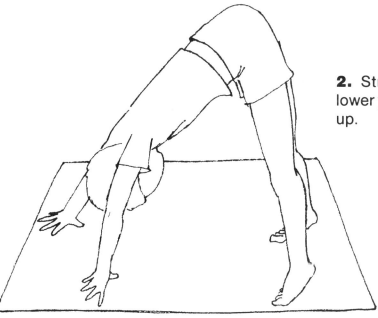

2. Straighten your legs and lower your head. Keep your heels up.

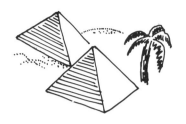

3. Lower your heels to the floor. Hold. Count 5.

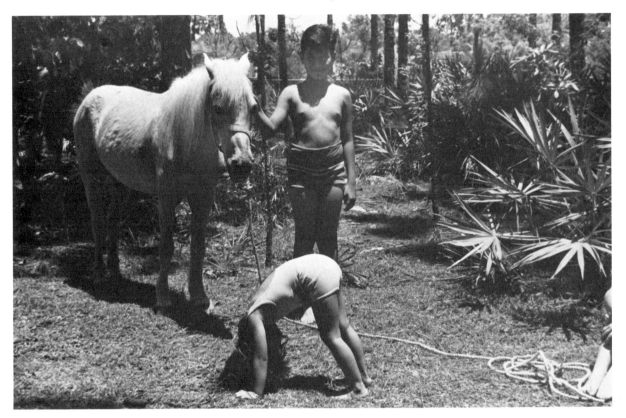

4. Slowly squat.

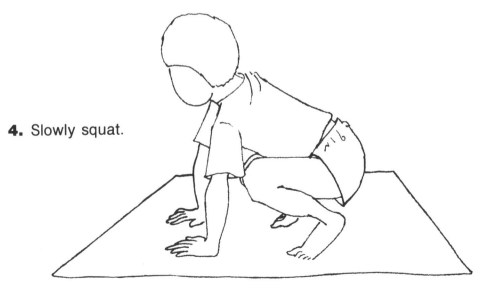

HOW TO DO THE EXERCISE:

If you cannot straighten your legs, practice with your knees bent. It may take one or two weeks for your legs to stretch enough to let your heels reach the floor. When you come back to the squatting position, raise your head very slowly.

After two weeks of counting 5, try for the count of 10. Do not go past the count of 10. Do the exercise twice.

WHAT THE EXERCISE DOES FOR YOU:

Stretches the back of your legs

Increases your energy

NOTE TO PARENTS AND TEACHERS:

Do not be disturbed if the child feels a slight pull in the back of his legs. Daily activities do not adequately stretch that part of the body.

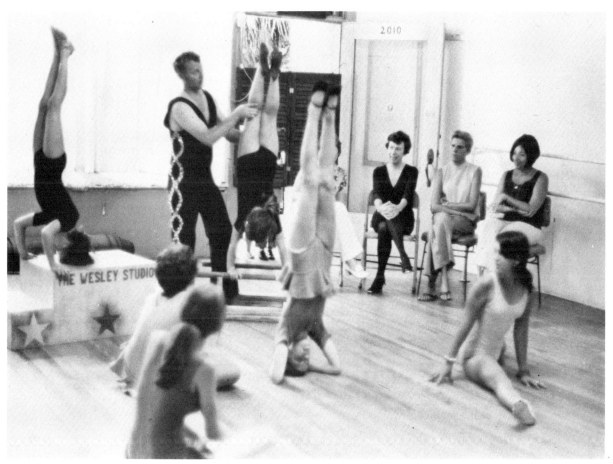

Acrobats learn yoga too.

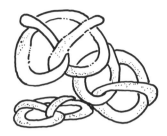

PRETZEL

●

1. Bend your right leg. Keep your knee on the floor. Bend your left leg. Hold your left ankle with both hands. Your feet should be touching.

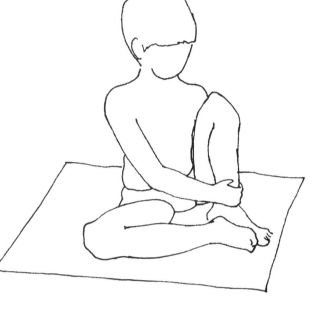

2. Lift your left foot and place it behind your right knee.

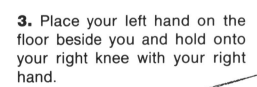

3. Place your left hand on the floor beside you and hold onto your right knee with your right hand.

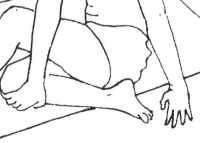

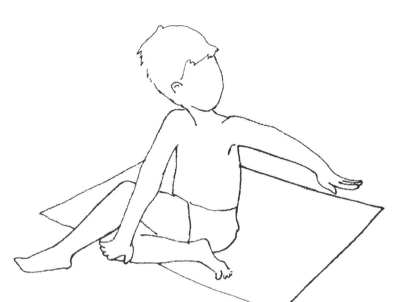

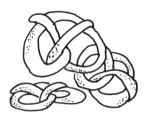

4. Bring your left arm straight out in front of your face, palm down. Slowly swing your left arm around to your left and turn your head to your left. Follow your arm with your eyes.

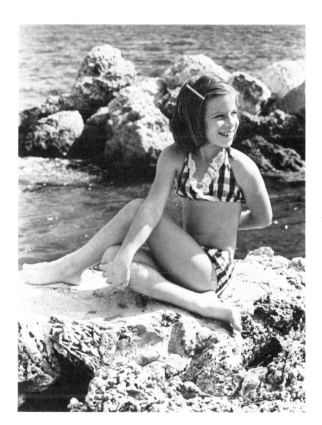

5. Bring your arm across your back. Hold. Count 10.

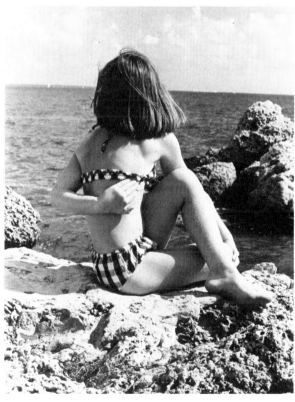

This is the way the exercise should look from the back.

143

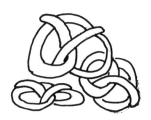

6. Slowly bring your head back to the front position, bring your arms to your sides, and place your hands on the floor.

7. Legs out. Rest.

8. Repeat on the other side, with your left knee on the floor.

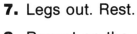

HOW TO DO THE EXERCISE:

If you find that you cannot grasp your knee, straighten your other leg. Do not be concerned if you cannot bring your arm all the way across your back. You may have to practice for a couple of weeks first.

After two weeks of counting 10, try for the count of 15. After four weeks of counting 15, try for the count of 20. Do this exercise twice.

WHAT THE EXERCISE DOES FOR YOU:

Improves your posture

Helps you grow straight and tall

NOTE TO PARENTS AND TEACHERS:

This exercise keeps the child's back limber by providing a spiral stretch for the spine. Very few yoga exercises do so. Since it is highly beneficial to stretch in this way, have the child do the exercise regularly.

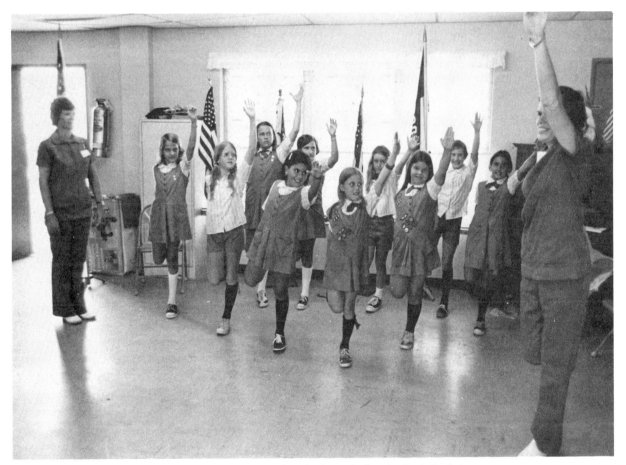

Girl Scouts are well trained. Yoga helps in their training.

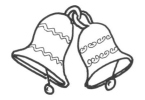

RINGING BELL

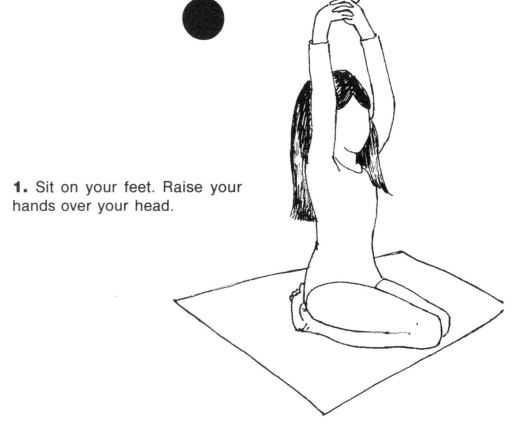

1. Sit on your feet. Raise your hands over your head.

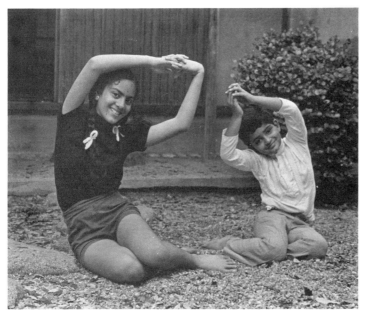

2. Sit to the left of your feet. Hold. Count 2. Sit to the right of your feet. Hold. Count 2. Swing from side to side 10 times (5 times to the left and 5 times to the right).

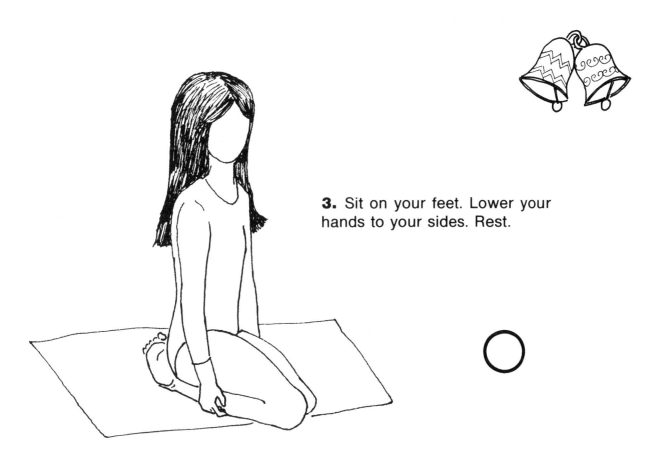

3. Sit on your feet. Lower your hands to your sides. Rest.

HOW TO DO THE EXERCISE:

As you sit to the left of your feet, swing your arms to the right. As you sit to the right of your feet, swing your arms to the left. Keep your back straight and use your back muscles to lift yourself up and over to each side. Pretend that you are holding a large bell and ringing it as you swing from side to side. Try to follow the same smooth rhythm all the way.

Do the exercise 10 times and rest. Do the exercise 10 times again.

WHAT THE EXERCISE DOES FOR YOU:

Strengthens your back muscles

Makes your legs feel loose so you can move around easily

NOTE TO PARENTS AND TEACHERS:

Try to have the child establish rhythm both in his breathing and in his body movements. He should pause only for a moment when he sits beside his feet. He can, if he likes, make the sounds of bells ringing. While having fun, he also improves his physical health.

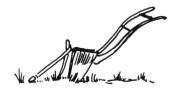

PLOW

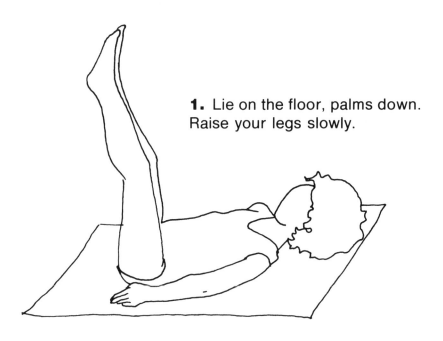

1. Lie on the floor, palms down. Raise your legs slowly.

2. Push your hands down against the floor. Raise your hips.

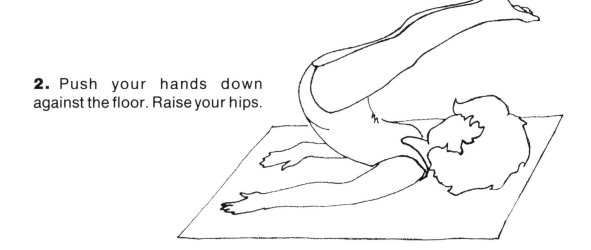

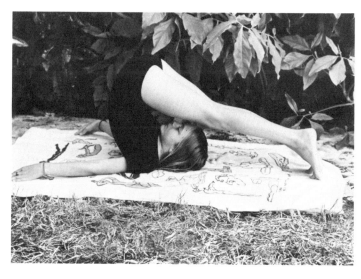

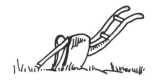

3. Very slowly, touch your toes to the floor in back of your head. Hold. Count 10.

4. Place your hands on top of your head. Hold. Count 10.

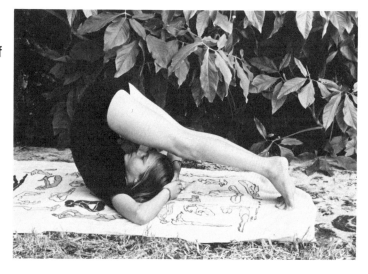

5. Bring your knees to your ears. Hold. Count 10.

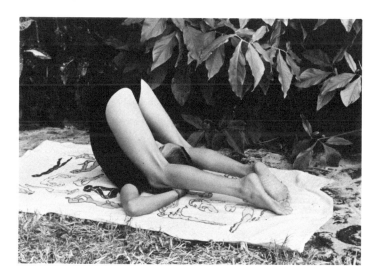

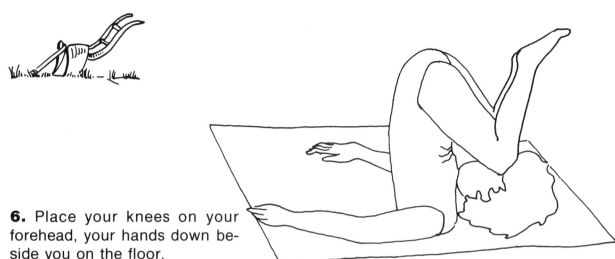

6. Place your knees on your forehead, your hands down beside you on the floor.

7. Roll your hips to the floor, knees close to your chest.

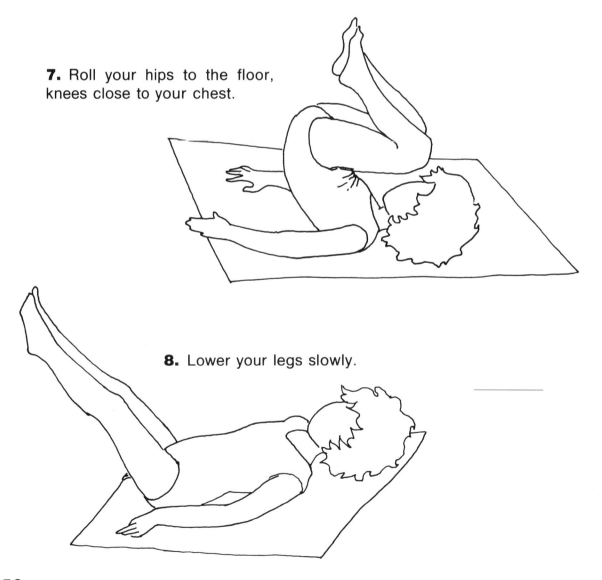

8. Lower your legs slowly.

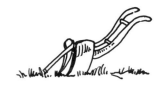

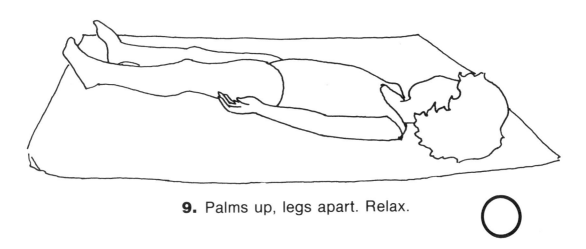

9. Palms up, legs apart. Relax.

HOW TO DO THE EXERCISE:

Be sure that you are ready for this exercise before you try it. If at the beginning your toes do not touch the floor behind you, just go as far as you can and hold that posture. You must not force your toes to touch the floor. It may take many weeks of practice before your back muscles stretch enough so that you can do the exercise comfortably.

After holding each position for the count of 10 for two weeks, try for the count of 15. Count 15 for four weeks. Then try for the count of 20. Do not go past the count of 20. Do the exercise twice.

WHAT THE EXERCISE DOES FOR YOU:

Strengthens your lower back and your stomach muscles

Keeps your back, neck, and spine loose

NOTE TO PARENTS AND TEACHERS:

The child must have a blanket or rug under his back, neck, and head. The Plow correlates well with two other yoga exercises: the Ballet Dancer and the Jelly Roll. To provide variety, have the child start with the Ballet Dancer (once on each side), then do the Plow and conclude with the Jelly Roll.

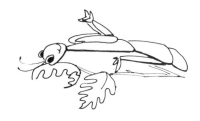

PRAYING MANTIS

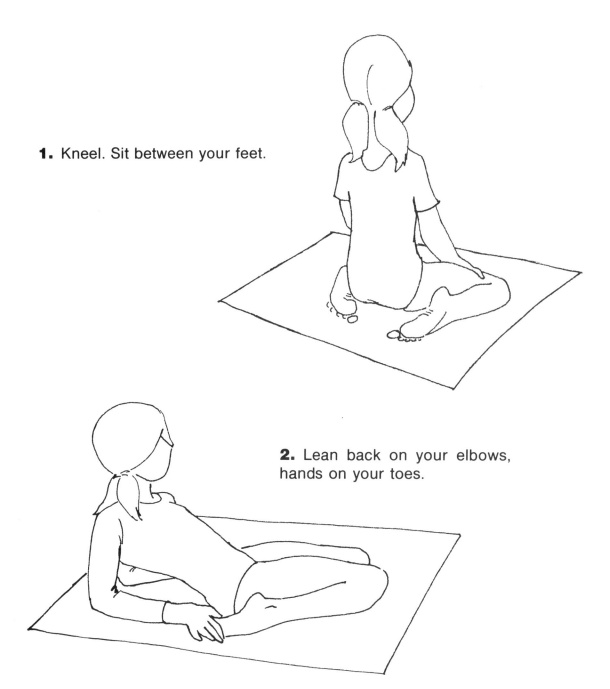

1. Kneel. Sit between your feet.

2. Lean back on your elbows, hands on your toes.

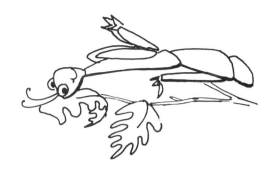

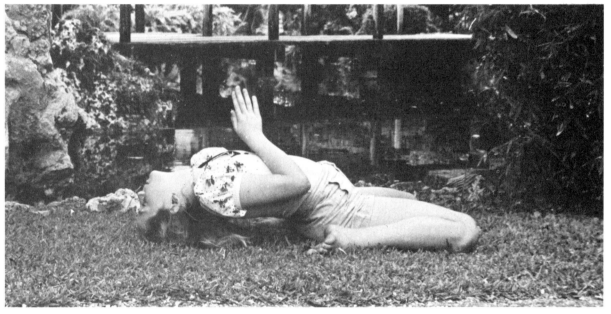

3. Rest your head on the floor. Point your chin straight up. Raise your back a little bit. Put the palms of your hands together as though you are praying. Hold. Count 10.

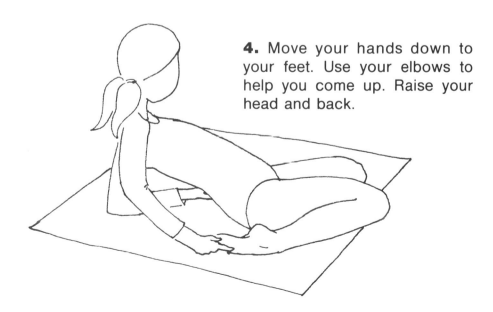

4. Move your hands down to your feet. Use your elbows to help you come up. Raise your head and back.

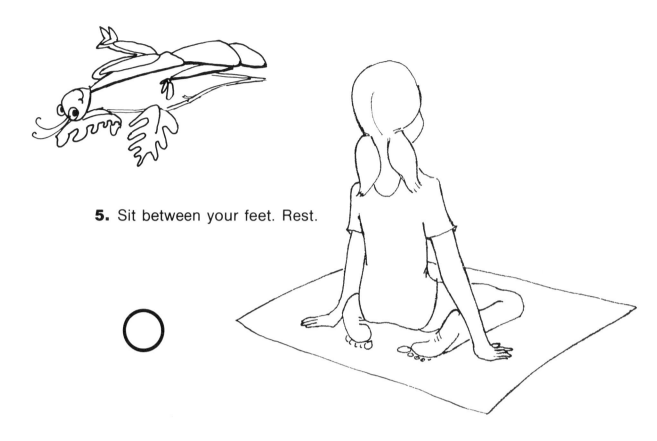

5. Sit between your feet. Rest.

HOW TO DO THE EXERCISE:

Be sure that you can sit comfortably before you try to lie down all the way. You may need one or two weeks to give your legs a chance to stretch. Remember to move very slowly as you go in and out of the exercise. After you have held the count of 10 for two weeks, try for the count of 15. Count 15 for four weeks. Then try for the count of 20. Do the exercise twice.

WHAT THE EXERCISE DOES FOR YOU:

Keeps your back and legs loose so you can move easily

NOTE TO PARENTS AND TEACHERS:

This is an advanced posture, requiring a great deal of preliminary flexibility in the back and legs. Caution children not to hurry into the exercise or out of it.

FULL LOCUST

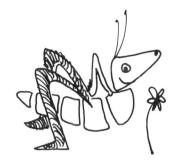

1. Lie on your tummy. Place your chin on the floor. Make fists, keeping your hands close to your body.

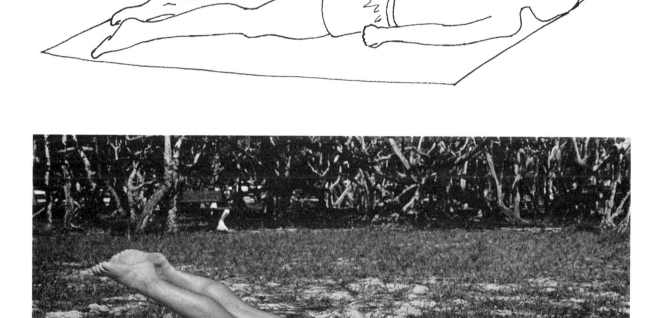

2. Press down hard with your fists. Raise both your legs slowly. Hold. Count 3.

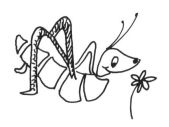

3. Lower your legs slowly. Turn your head to the side. Relax.

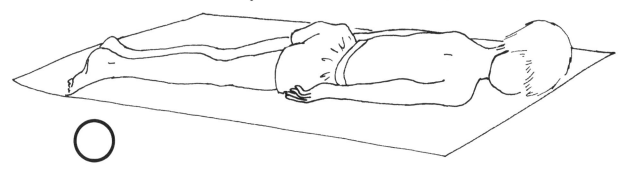

HOW TO DO THE EXERCISE:

Remember to raise and lower your legs slowly. Do not expect to raise them very high when you begin. As you raise them, put your weight on your hands, chest, and chin.

After you have held the count of 3 for four weeks, try for the count of 5. Do not go past the count of 5. Do the exercise twice.

WHAT THIS EXERCISE DOES FOR YOU:

Strengthens your arms and lower back

NOTE TO PARENTS AND TEACHERS:

Do not allow the child to strain as he holds his legs up. It is harder for him to raise both legs than to raise one at a time, as in the Half Locust; but raising both legs is highly beneficial for him as it helps to firm the muscles of his thighs, hips, back, and buttocks. Counting 5 slowly is sufficient time to hold this exercise.

HEAD STAND

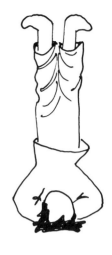

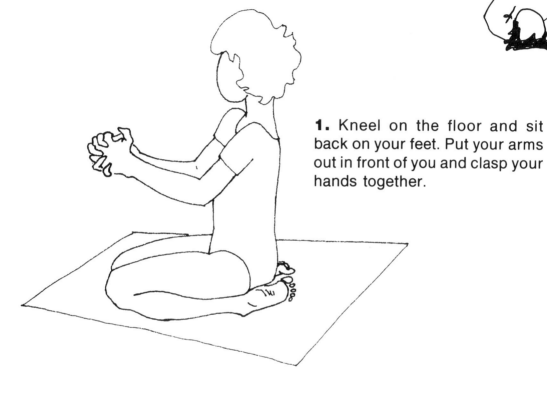

1. Kneel on the floor and sit back on your feet. Put your arms out in front of you and clasp your hands together.

2. Lower your arms to the floor. Bend your elbows. Lean forward.

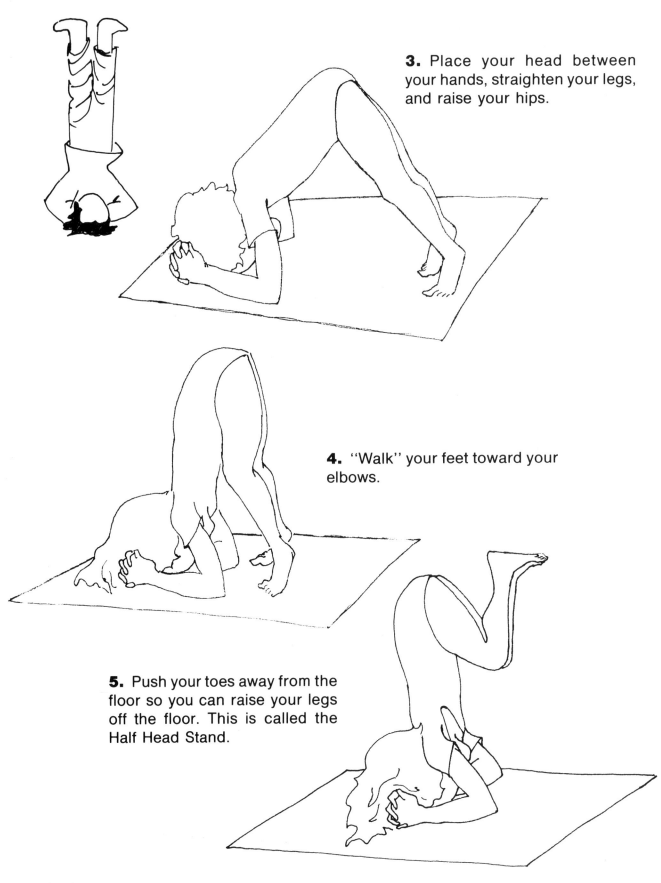

3. Place your head between your hands, straighten your legs, and raise your hips.

4. "Walk" your feet toward your elbows.

5. Push your toes away from the floor so you can raise your legs off the floor. This is called the Half Head Stand.

158

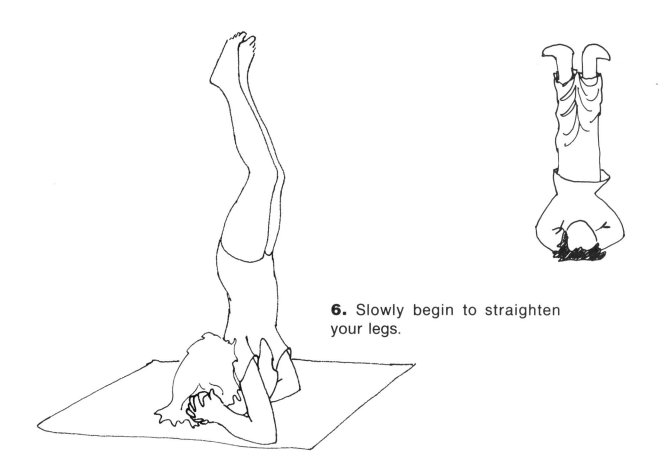

6. Slowly begin to straighten your legs.

7. Get your legs to stand straight up in the air. Hold. Count 10. This is the Head Stand.

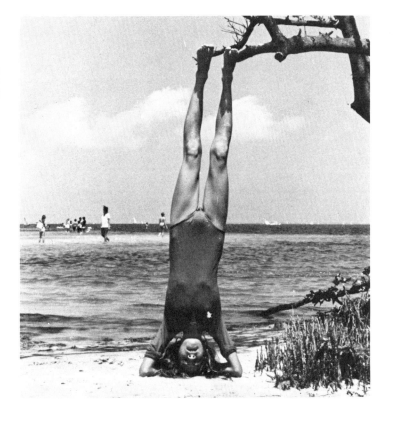

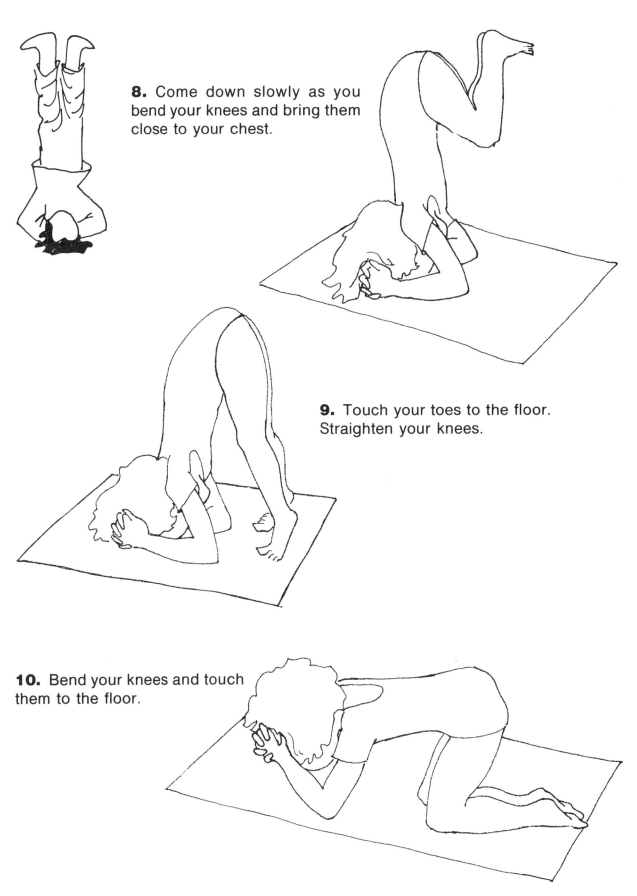

8. Come down slowly as you bend your knees and bring them close to your chest.

9. Touch your toes to the floor. Straighten your knees.

10. Bend your knees and touch them to the floor.

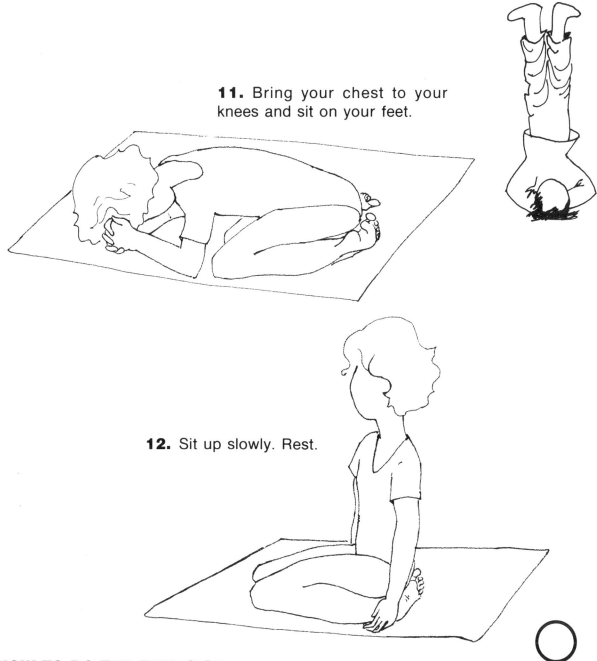

11. Bring your chest to your knees and sit on your feet.

12. Sit up slowly. Rest.

HOW TO DO THE EXERCISE:

After you lower your arms to the floor (figure 2), cross them and hold your elbows. First, place your right hand on your left elbow. Then place your left hand on your right elbow. Look at the drawing of the arms. It will help you. Now straighten your arms without moving your elbows. Clasp your hands together.

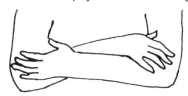

Practice the Half Head Stand (figure 5) for two or three weeks before you try to raise your legs up in the air and go into the Head Stand. If your neck should feel uncomfortable in either of the positions, come out s-l-o-w-l-y. Do not hold the position.

When you finish figure 11, you must rest. Count 10 before you sit up. Be sure you do this. You can get dizzy if you sit up too quickly.

Hold the count of 10 for four weeks. Then try for the count of 20. Hold the count of 20 for four weeks. Then try for the count of 30. Do not go past the count of 30. Do the exercise once.

WHAT THE EXERCISE DOES FOR YOU:

Helps you think better

Gives you energy

NOTE TO PARENTS AND TEACHERS:

The Head Stand is invigorating, but the child must be careful in performing it. Should he ever experience discomfort in his neck, he must come down immediately, although in gradual steps. This cannot be emphasized too strongly. He can then try the exercise again.

He should not do this exercise directly after eating, nor should he do it before bed. Neither his stomach nor his sleep will be disturbed, however, if he reserves some time to practice after school or before dinner.

Note that both the Head Stand and the Hand Stand exercise are given in this program. The Head Stand is less difficult to accomplish and should therefore be learned first.

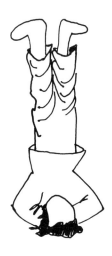

CAMEL

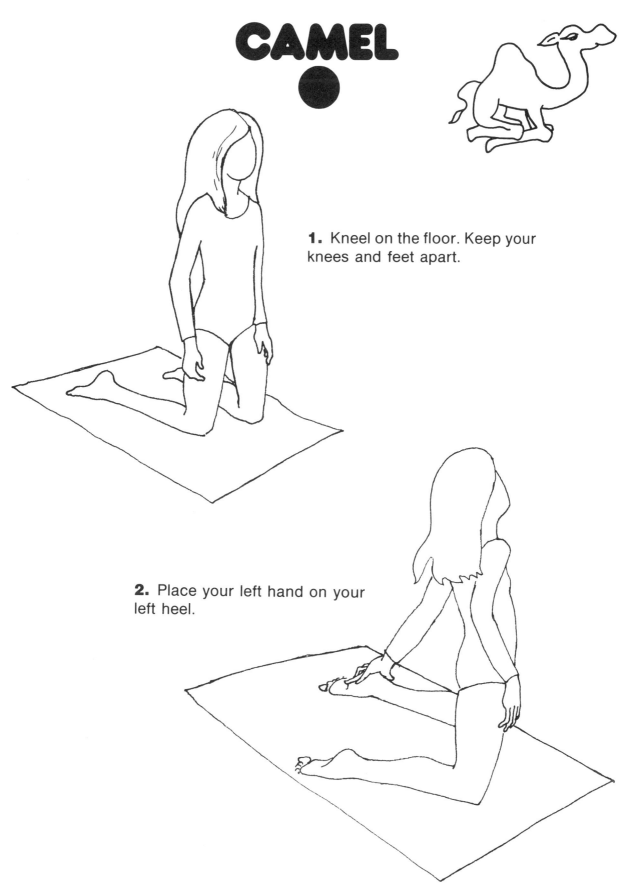

1. Kneel on the floor. Keep your knees and feet apart.

2. Place your left hand on your left heel.

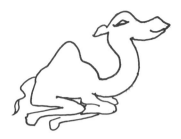

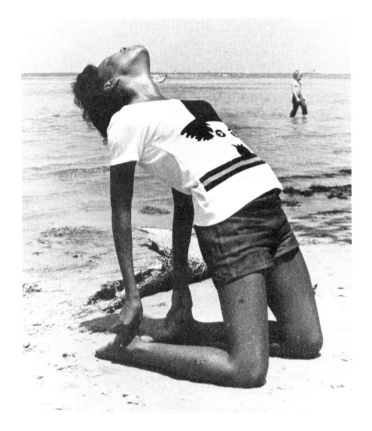

3. Place your right hand on your right heel. Push your chest up and let your head drop back. Hold. Count 5.

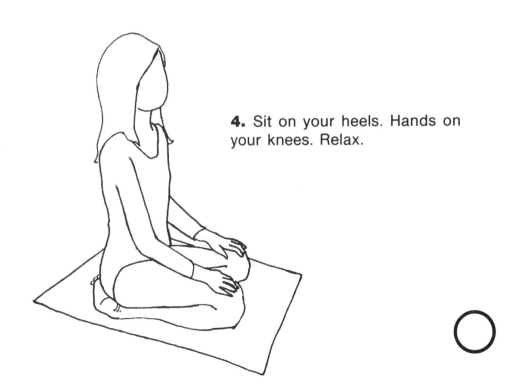

4. Sit on your heels. Hands on your knees. Relax.

HOW TO DO THE EXERCISE:

If you cannot do the exercise, practice stretching back with one hand at a time. Be sure that you are kneeling on something soft.

After you have held the count of 5 for two weeks, try for the count of 10. Count 10 for four weeks. Then try for the count of 20. Do not go past the count of 20. Do the exercise twice.

WHAT THE EXERCISE DOES FOR YOU:

Keeps your back loose

Relaxes your neck

Helps you think better

NOTE TO PARENTS AND TEACHERS:

This exercise requires considerable flexibility to begin with. Caution the child to refrain from forcing the hold position.

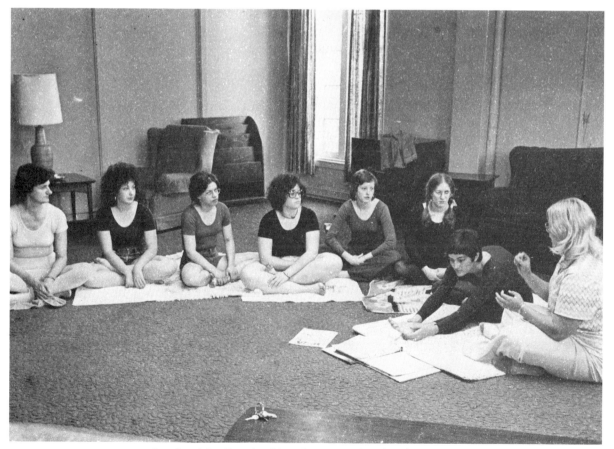

A school for the deaf teaches yoga by sign language.

BOW

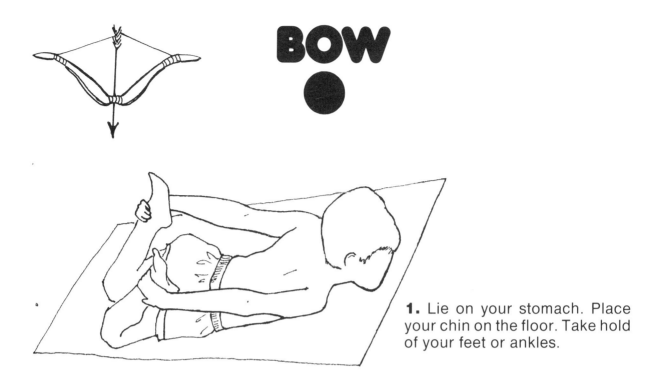

1. Lie on your stomach. Place your chin on the floor. Take hold of your feet or ankles.

2. Pull your legs back. This will raise your knees and chest. Hold. Count 3.

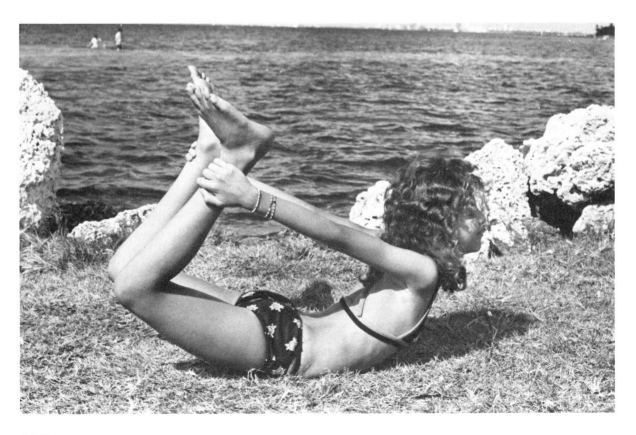

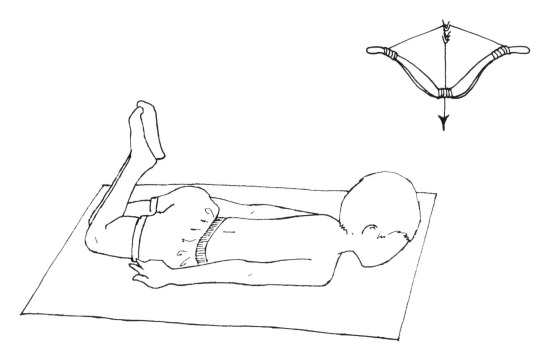

3. Let go of your legs, lower your knees, and bring your chest and chin to the floor. Place your hands at your sides.

4. Straighten your legs. Turn your head to the side and rest.

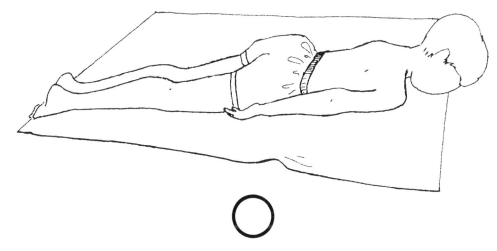

HOW TO DO THE EXERCISE:

To get your chest and knees off the floor, keep your arms straight and pull your legs back slowly. Be careful. Do not use too much force. This exercise is hard to do. Rest every time you do it. After you have held the count of 3 for two weeks, try for the count of 5. Do not go past the count of 5. Do the exercise twice.

WHAT THE EXERCISE DOES FOR YOU:

Strengthens your back

NOTE TO PARENTS AND TEACHERS:

The Bow is a demanding exercise. Make sure the child does not strain himself as he tries to do it. If he can only raise his knees one or two inches from the floor, consider that adequate. Once his back muscles strengthen, he will be able to raise his knees higher. He does not need strength in his arms to raise his knees. The strength must be in his lower back and legs. Tell him not to pull forward with his arms, but to keep them straight as he slowly pulls his legs back.

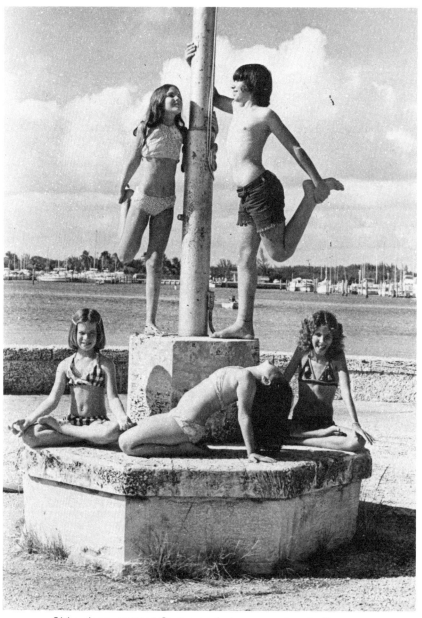

Ship ahoy, mates! Come and share our fun in the sun.

TUMMY LIFT

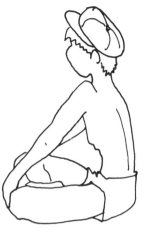

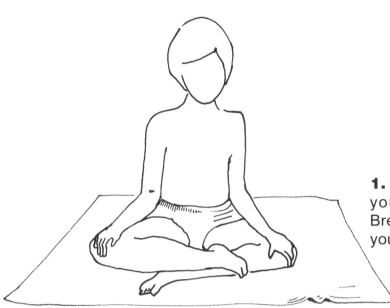

1. Sit with your legs crossed, your hands on your knees. Breathe out all the air inside of you.

2. Pull your tummy in and up. Hold. Count 3 silently.

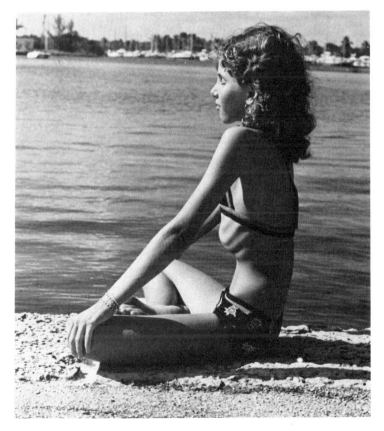

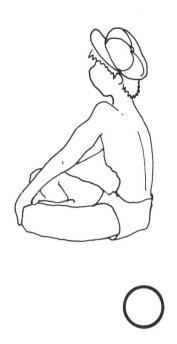

3. Push ("pop") your tummy out.

4. Breathe in. Relax.

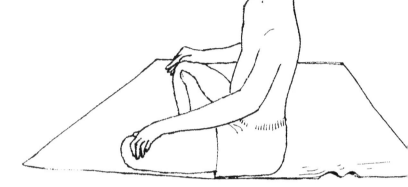

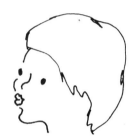

HOW TO DO THE EXERCISE:

Breathe out as much air as you can by puckering your lips and slowly whistling.

As you pull your tummy in, press your hands down on your knees. As you push your tummy out, relax your hands. If it is not comfortable for you to place your hands on your knees because your knees are too high, do the Tummy Lift with your hands on the floor behind you.

Wait until you push your tummy out before you breathe in. Do the exercise 5 times. Rest. Do the exercise 5 times again. You should never do this exercise immediately after eating. It is best to wait two or three hours.

WHAT THE EXERCISE DOES FOR YOU:

Tightens your tummy muscles

Keeps you from being constipated

NOTE TO PARENTS AND TEACHERS:

No other yoga exercise duplicates this one. It massages and strengthens the child's internal organs. When you feel that he can do this exercise easily, have him try something more advanced. Tell him not to breathe in until he has achieved three Tummy Lifts.

BRIDGE

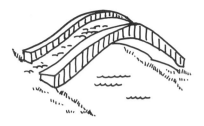

1. Lie on your back. Bend your knees. Take hold of your ankles.

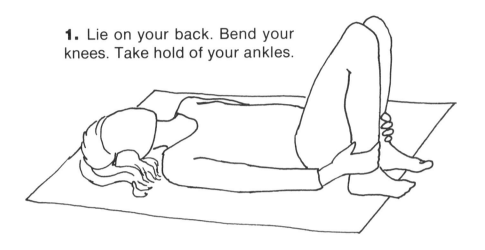

2. Push your back up. Hold. Count to 5.

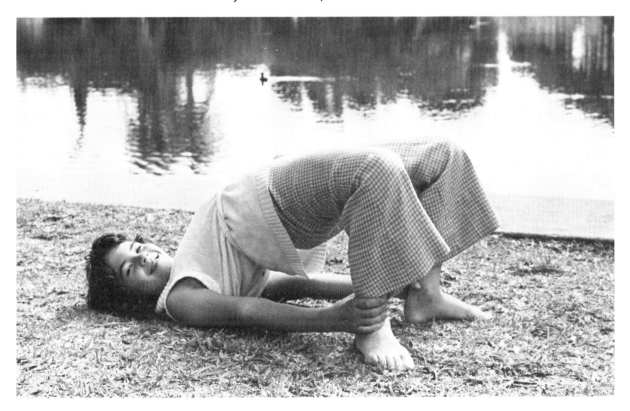

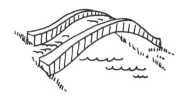

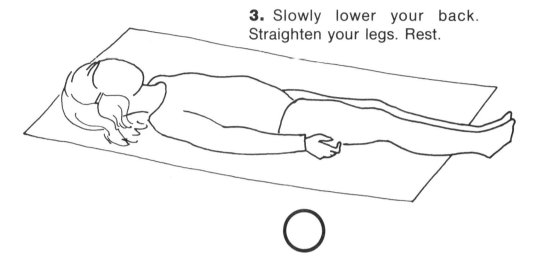

3. Slowly lower your back. Straighten your legs. Rest.

HOW TO DO THE EXERCISE:

Raise and lower your back slowly. Use a soft cover on the floor. If after four weeks you feel that you can hold the count of 5 easily, try for the count of 10. Do not go past the count of 10. Do the exercise twice.

WHAT THE EXERCISE DOES FOR YOU:

Strengthens your back and leg muscles and gives them good movement

NOTE TO PARENTS AND TEACHERS:

Do not be surprised to find that some children cannot accomplish the exercise successfully at first. An initial amount of muscle strength is required to achieve the posture.

WHEEL

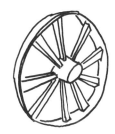

1. Lie on your back. Bend your knees. Place your hands near your ears with your fingers turned toward your shoulders.

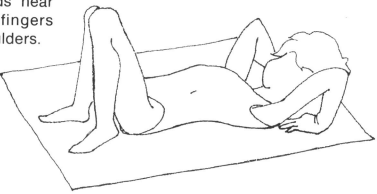

2. Push down with your hands. Raise your back. Hold. Count 5.

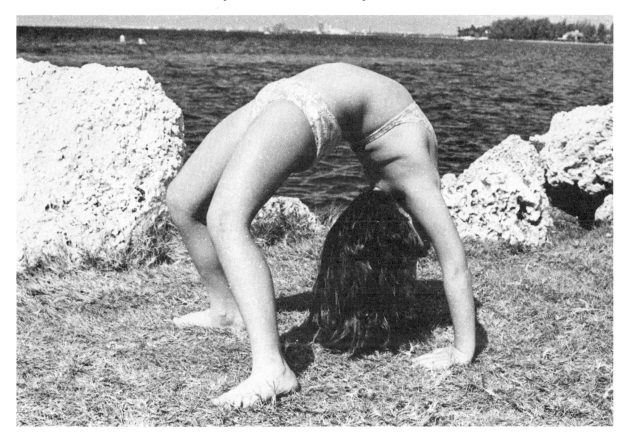

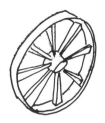

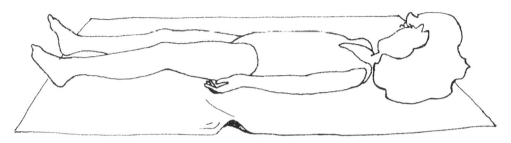

3. Come down slowly. Lie flat on your back, with your arms at your sides, palms turned up. Keep your legs apart. Rest.

HOW TO DO THE EXERCISE:

This is a very hard exercise to do. You must be sure to rest every time you finish it.

If you cannot straighten your arms, you will not be able to raise your head from the floor. Be content with raising your back and keeping your head on the floor. As you continue to practice, your arms will get stronger and you will be able to raise your back and head from the floor. After you have held the count of 5 for four weeks, try for the count of 10. Do not go past the count of 10. Do the exercise twice.

WHAT THE EXERCISE DOES FOR YOU:

Gives your brain energy and helps you think better

Strengthens your arms

Keeps your back loose

NOTE TO PARENTS AND TEACHERS:

Caution the child to refrain from exerting himself too much.

SALUTE TO THE SUN

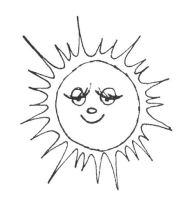

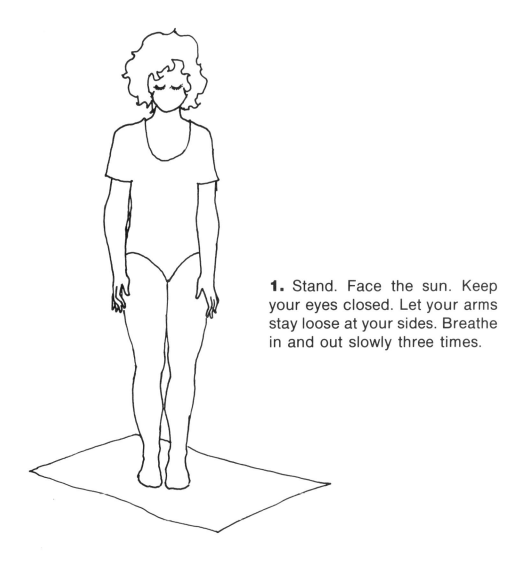

1. Stand. Face the sun. Keep your eyes closed. Let your arms stay loose at your sides. Breathe in and out slowly three times.

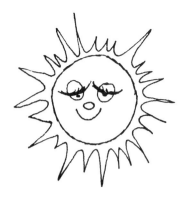

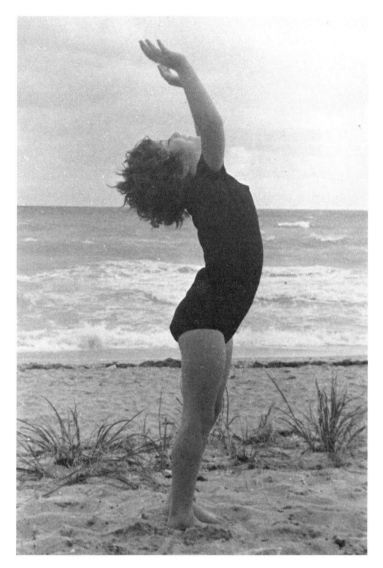

2. Breathe in. Keep on breathing in as you stretch your arms up and bend back.

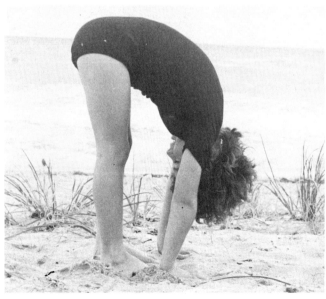

3. Breathe out. Keep on breathing out while you slowly bend forward and bring your hands to the floor.

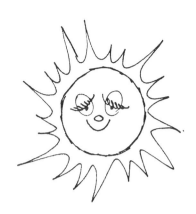

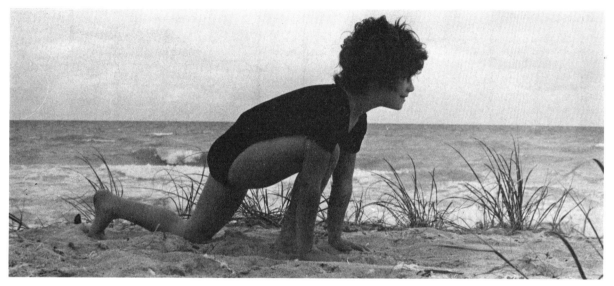

4. Breathe in. Keep on breathing in but raise your head and stretch your left leg behind you. Your right knee should now touch your chest.

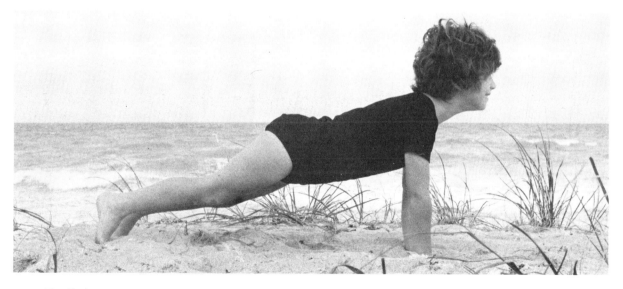

5. Bring your right leg to your left leg. Hold your breath. Count 4 silently.

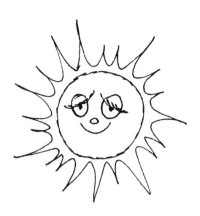

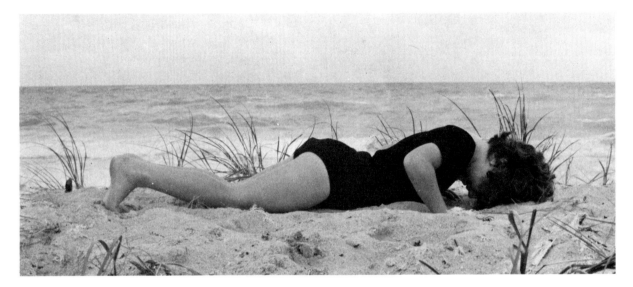

6. Breathe out. Keep on breathing out while you slowly bend your elbows and place your head, chest, and knees on the floor.

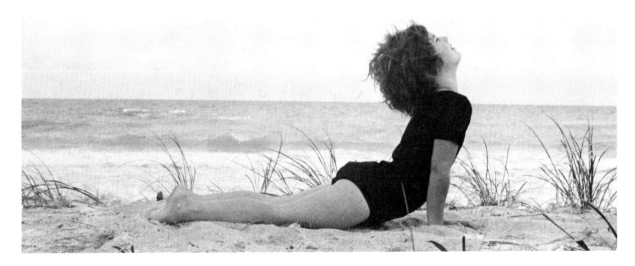

7. Breathe in. Keep on breathing in while you straighten your arms and raise your head and chest. Do not move your hands.

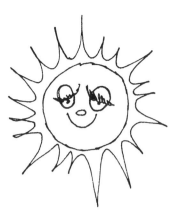

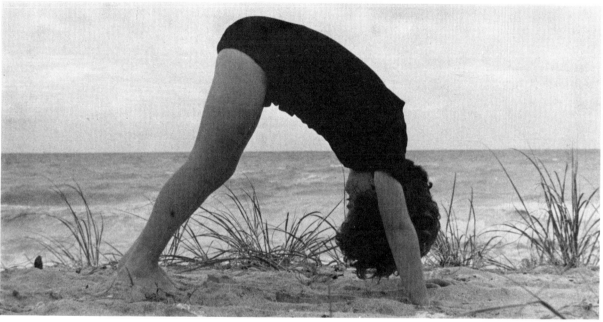

8. Breathe out. Keep on breathing out as you place the soles of your feet on the floor and you raise your hips and lower your head. Do not move your hands.

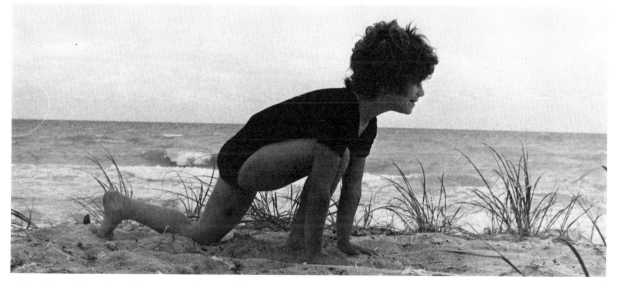

9. Breathe in. Keep on breathing in as you bring your right knee to your chest.

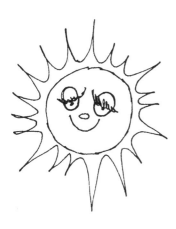

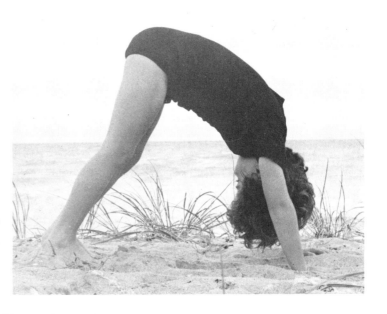

10. Breathe out. Keep on breathing out as you bring your left foot to your right foot. Raise your hips and lower your head.

11. Breathe in. Keep on breathing in as you stand and you raise your arms and put your head back.

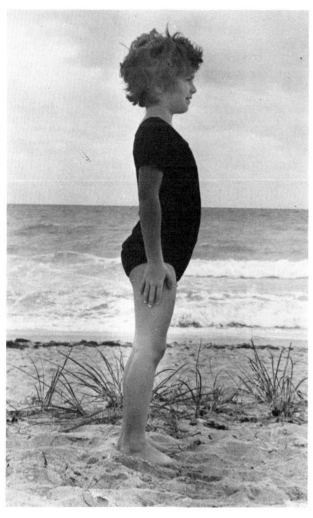

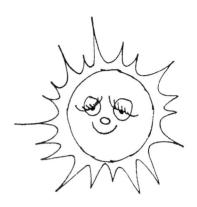

12. Breathe out. Keep on breathing out as you bring your arms to your sides. Rest.

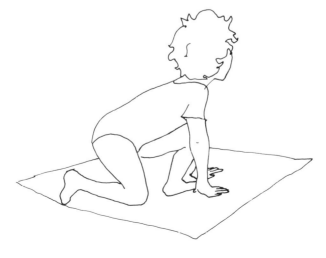

HOW TO DO THE EXERCISE:

Do the exercise smoothly. Do not rush from one step to the other. Take your time. Hold each position for the count of four. When you finish doing the exercise once (figure 9), do it again, but this time put your right leg behind you and let your left leg touch your chest. See the illustration below.

WHAT THE EXERCISE DOES FOR YOU:

Helps your whole body grow tall and straight

NOTE TO PARENTS AND TEACHERS:

This is the only yoga exercise that moves continuously from one position to the next. None of the steps are held for an extended period of time. There is only a 3- or 4-second hold, a fleeting pause between the steps. This very brief pause does not interfere with the flow of the movements.

After the children learn to do the exercise correctly, the tempo may be slightly increased. However, keep in mind the fact that yoga is not a form of calisthenics and is done with the expenditure of a minimum amount of energy. At no time should a child feel exhausted after completing a yoga exercise.

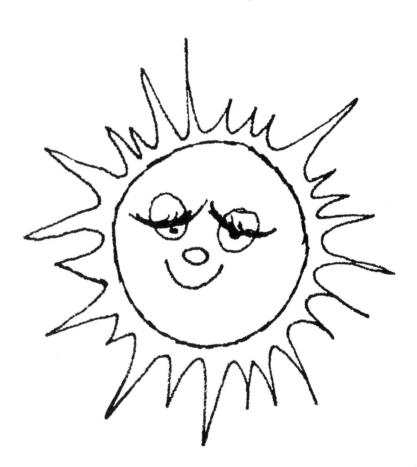

PECKING CHICKEN

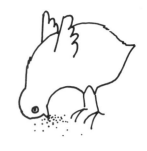

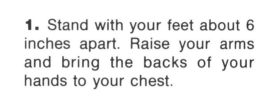

1. Stand with your feet about 6 inches apart. Raise your arms and bring the backs of your hands to your chest.

2. Slowly swing your hands behind you and clasp them.

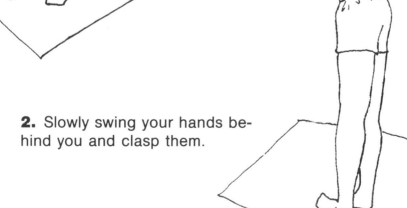

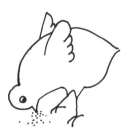

3. Bend back slowly. Hold. Count 3.

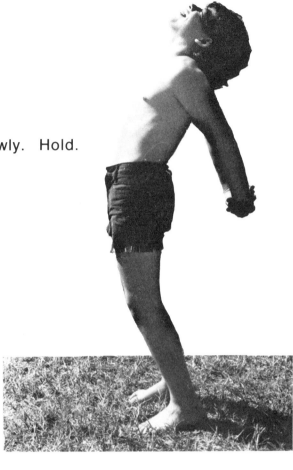

4. Bend forward slowly. Hold. Count 5.

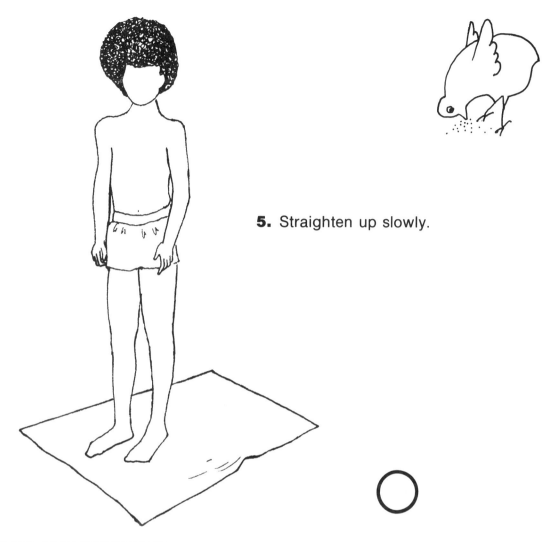

5. Straighten up slowly.

HOW TO DO THE EXERCISE:

Try to keep your arms as high as you can when you bend backward and forward. Do not be concerned if your arms do not go very high at first. For better balance, keep your eyes open.

After two weeks, raise the backward count to 5 and the forward count to 10. After four weeks, raise the forward count to 15 and keep the backward count of 5. Hold these counts for four weeks. Now keep the backward count of 5 but raise the forward count to 20.

WHAT THE EXERCISE DOES FOR YOU:

Gives you good posture

Gives you more energy

NOTE TO PARENTS AND TEACHERS:

This is a pick-me-up exercise. It diminishes fatigue and helps the child feel alert. It also keeps the back and neck flexible and relaxed.

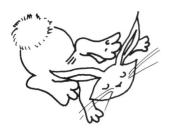

BUNNY TAIL

●

1. Lie on your back, legs apart.

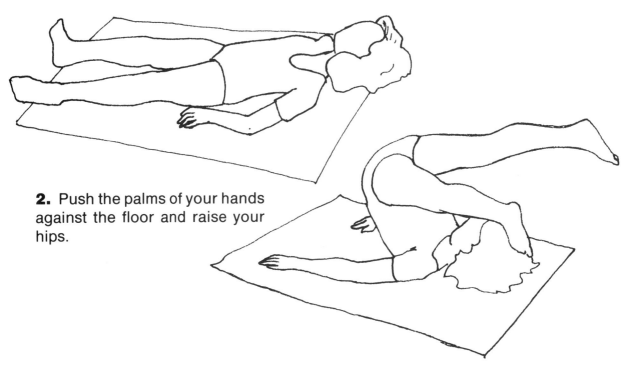

2. Push the palms of your hands against the floor and raise your hips.

3. Touch your toes to the floor behind you and keep them there with your hands. Hold. Count 10.

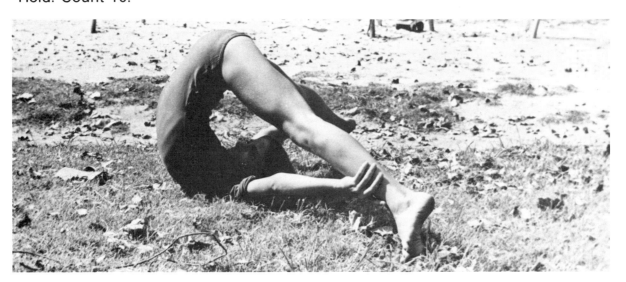

4. Bring your hands back to the floor beside you and roll forward slowly. Rest.

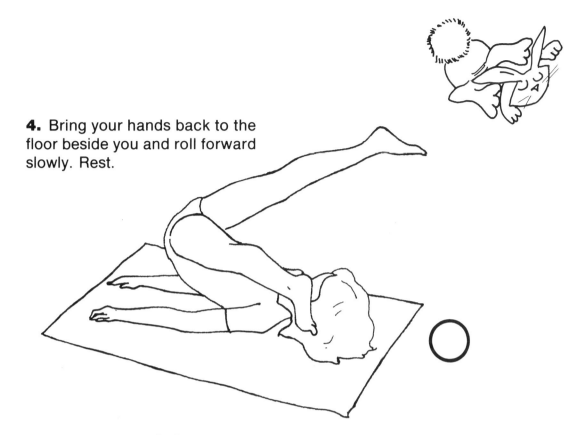

HOW TO DO THE EXERCISE:

Do not do this exercise on a hard floor. Be sure that you are lying on a rug or a blanket.

Try to keep your knees straight. After you have held the count of 10 for two weeks, try for the count of 15. Count 15 for four weeks. Then try for the count of 20. Do the exercise twice.

WHAT THE EXERCISE DOES FOR YOU:

Stretches the backs of your legs

Keeps your spine and neck loose so they can move easily

Gives you energy

NOTE TO PARENTS AND TEACHERS:

Perfecting this exercise calls for a great deal of flexibility in the back. If the child cannot reach the floor with his toes, tell him to go only as far as he can and hold the position he is in.

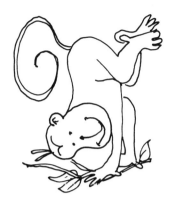

HAND STAND

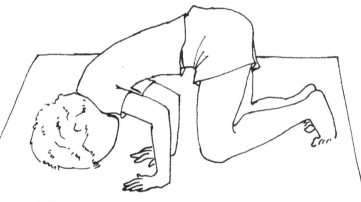

1. Kneel. Turn your toes forward. Place your head and hands on the floor.

2. Push your toes away from the floor so you can raise your legs off the floor. Rest your knees on the backs of your arms. This is called the Half Hand Stand.

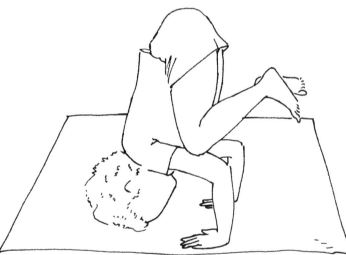

3. When you feel that you have your balance, begin to straighten your legs.

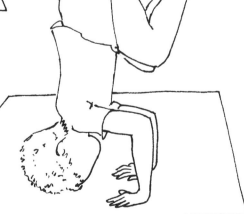

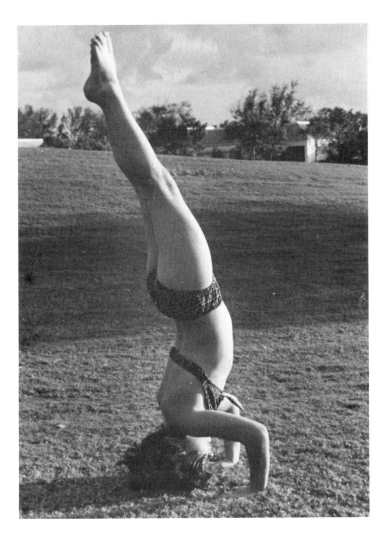

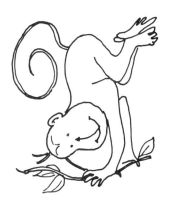

4. Get your legs to stand straight up in the air. Hold. Count 10. This is the Hand Stand.

5. Bend your knees. Bring them close to your chest. Start to bring your feet down.

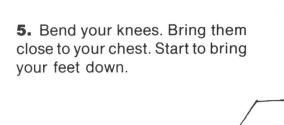

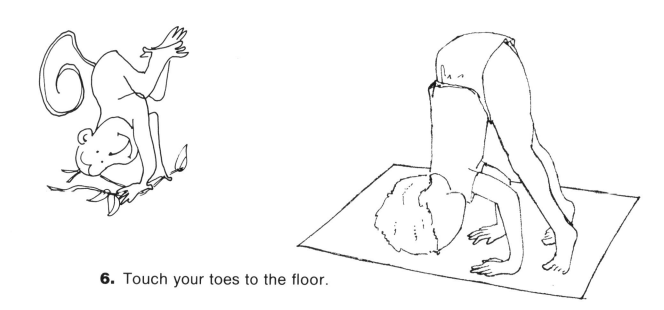

6. Touch your toes to the floor.

7. Kneel. Bring your chest close to the floor and sit on your feet. Rest.

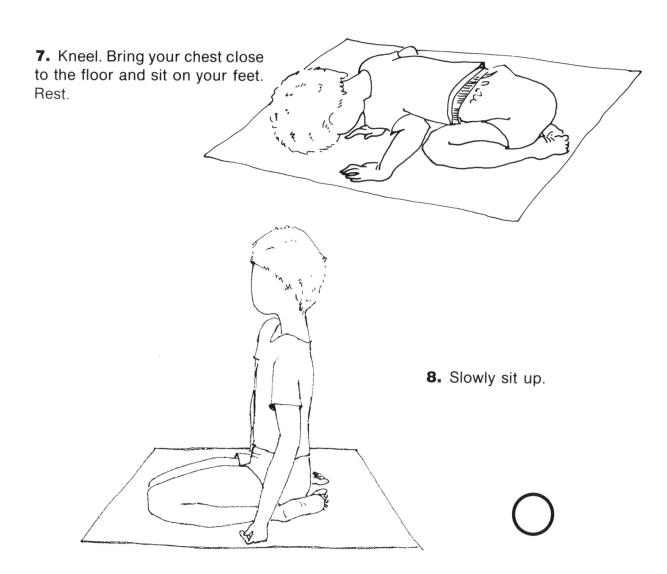

8. Slowly sit up.

HOW TO DO THE EXERCISE:

Practice the Half Hand Stand for two or three weeks before you try to raise your legs up in the air and go into the Hand Stand. If your neck should feel uncomfortable, do not hold this position. Come out s-l-o-w-l-y.

When you finish figure 7, you must rest. Count 10 before you sit up. Be sure you do this. You can get dizzy if you sit up too quickly.

Hold the count of 10 for four weeks. Then try for the count of 20. Hold the count of 20 for four weeks, then try for the count of 30. Do not go past the count of 30. Do the exercise once.

WHAT THE EXERCISE DOES FOR YOU:

Wakes up your mind so you can think better

Makes your arms and neck strong

NOTE TO PARENTS AND TEACHERS:

Caution the child to proceed very slowly and carefully as he practices the Hand Stand, holding it for just a few seconds when he is first learning it. Do not at any time let him hold the exercise for more than 30 seconds.

If he should ever experience discomfort in his neck, tell him to come down immediately, but in gradual steps. This cannot be emphasized too strongly. He can then try the exercise again.

Do not let the child do this exercise directly after eating or before going to bed.

Note that the Hand Stand exercise and the Head Stand exercise are similar in benefits, but the Hand Stand exercise is more difficult to accomplish and should not be done until the Head Stand exercise is perfected.

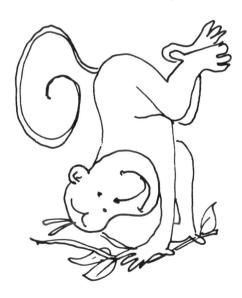

SPECIAL PROBLEMS

SCALP

Bridge	171
Hand Stand	188
Head Stand	157
Pecking Chicken	183
Pyramid	139
Rag Doll	30
Rocking Horse	93
Royal Hen	100
Salute to the Sun	175
Wheel	173

SHOULDERS

Back Scratch	78
Bow	166
Bridge	171
Candle	104
Cobra	114
Happy Feet	39
Pecking Chicken	183
Plow	148
Rocking Horse	93
Royal Hen	100
Salute to the Sun	175
Slide	123
Star	98
Twinkle Toes	95
Wheel	173

SLEEP

Balloon

Curling Leaf	80
Giraffe	42
Kitty Cat	36
Nosey Clown	132
Pretty Eyes	45
Rag Doll	30
Sleeper	50

SPINE

Ballet Dancer	82
Bow	166
Bridge	171
Camel	163
Cat	108
Cobra	114
Curling Leaf	80
Eagle Spread	85
Full Locust	155
Happy Feet	39
Half Locust	88
Jelly Roll	69
Kitty Cat	36
Pecking Chicken	183
Plow	148
Praying Mantis	152
Pretzel	142
Pyramid	139
Rabbit Sit	91
Rag Doll	30
Rocking Horse	93
Royal Hen	100
Salute to the Sun	175

Star	98
Twig	62
Twinkle Toes	95
Wheel	173

THIGHS

Bow	
Bridge	166
Camel	171
Cat	163
Curling Leaf	108
Eagle Spread	80
Frog	85
Full Locust	48
Half Locust	155
Lotus Bud	88
Lotus Flower	102
Octopus	129
Praying Mantis	136
Pretzel	152
Rabbit Sit	142
Ringing Bell	91
Salute to the Sun	146
Seesaw	175
Star	120
Stork	98
Strong Man	118
Tailor	33
Tree	52
Twig	62
Twinkle Toes	95

THROAT

Lion	60
Candle	104

TOES

Fly Away Bird	126
Octopus	136
Pretzel	142
Praying Mantis	152
Star	98
Strong Man	33
Twinkle Toes	95

TUMMY

Candle	104
Plow	148
Ringing Bell	146
Seesaw	120
Tummy Lift	169

WAIST

Pecking Chicken	183
Pretzel	142
Rag Doll	30
Royal Hen	100
Salute to the Sun	175
Triangle	54
Tummy Lift	169

WEIGHT

Note: Correct eating habits must go along with these exercises.

Balloon	74	Half Locust	88
Bow	166	Plow	148
Candle	104		

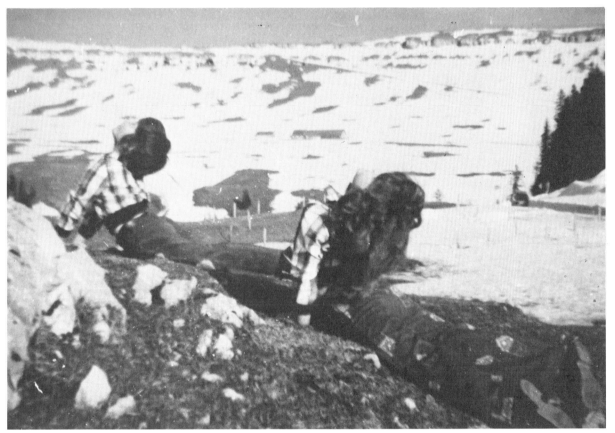

Yoga can be done anywhere. Here it is done on a snow covered mountain in Switzerland.

INDEX OF EXERCISES

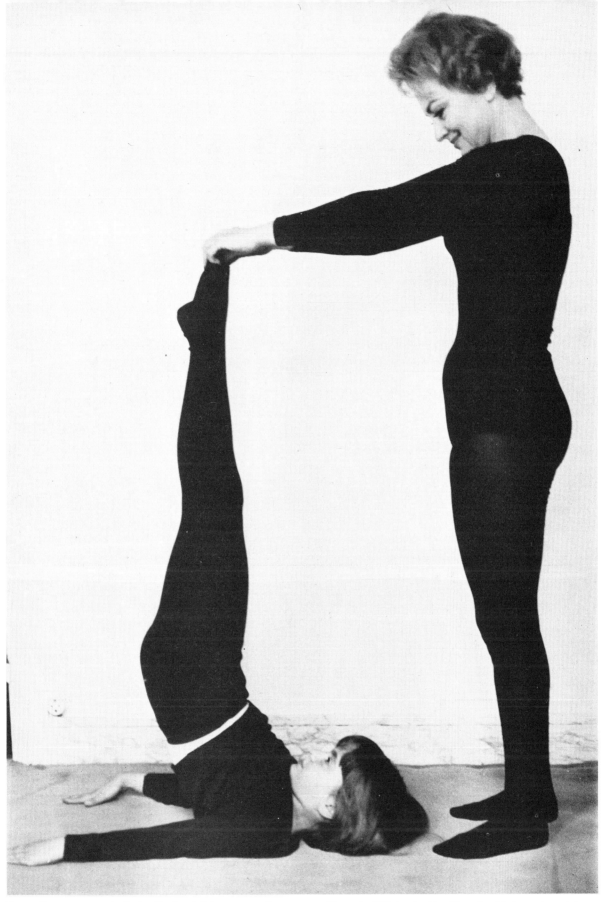

Sometimes parents help their children practice yoga. Here is Olivia de Havilland with her daughter Gisele. *(Photograph by Araldo Crollalanza)*

EXE CISE C A T

Keep a record of the exercises you do every day.

MONDAY	TUESDAY	WEDNESDAY	THURSDAY	FRIDAY	SATURDAY	SUNDAY

MONDAY	TUESDAY	WEDNESDAY	THURSDAY	FRIDAY	SATURDAY	SUNDAY

MONDAY	TUESDAY	WEDNESDAY	THURSDAY	FRIDAY	SATURDAY	SUNDAY

MONDAY	TUESDAY	WEDNESDAY	THURSDAY	FRIDAY	SATURDAY	SUNDAY

MONDAY	TUESDAY	WEDNESDAY	THURSDAY	FRIDAY	SATURDAY	SUNDAY

MONDAY	TUESDAY	WEDNESDAY	THURSDAY	FRIDAY	SATURDAY	SUNDAY

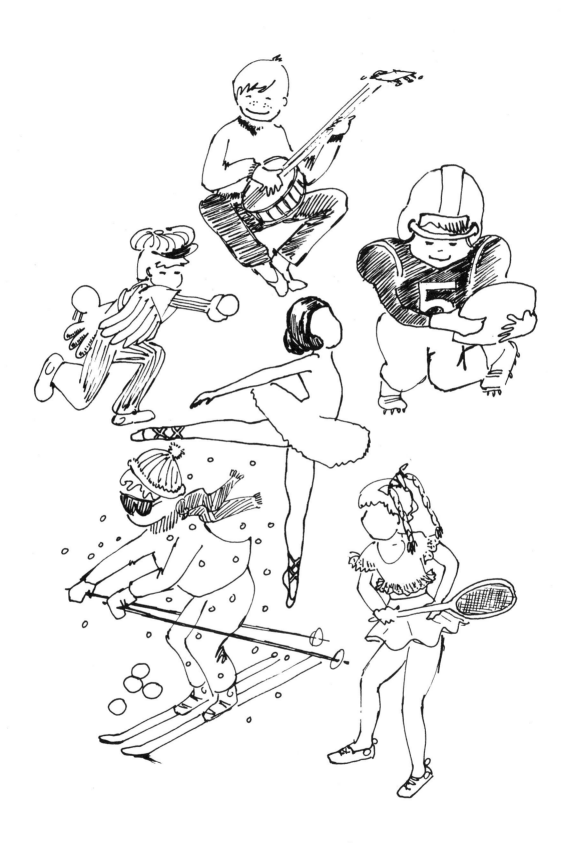